Generation V

The Complete Guide
to Going, Being, and Staying
Vegan
as a Teenager

Claire Askew

Generation **V**

The Complete Guide
to Going, Being, and Staying
Vegan
as a Teenager

Claire Askew

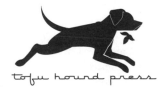

DISCLAIMER: Though this book has been thoroughly researched, the opinions herein are offered for educational and entertainment purposes only. Before any change in diet, readers should consult a physician or nutritionist. Although the author and publisher have made every effort to ensure the accuracy and completeness of information contained in this book, we assume no responsibility for errors, inaccuracies, omissions, or any inconsistency herein.

Generation V: The Complete Guide to Going, Being, and Staying Vegan as a Teenager © Claire Askew 2011
This edition © PM Press 2011

All rights reserved. No part of this book may be transmitted by any means without permission in writing from the publisher.

ISBN: 978-1-60486-338-3

Library of Congress Control Number: 2010927787

Cover design by Tofu Hound and John Yates/stealworks.com
Interior design by JBHR

PM Press
PO Box 23912
Oakland, CA 94623
www.pmpress.org

Printed by the Employee Owners of Thomson-Shore in Dexter, Michigan.
www.thomsonshore.com
Printed in the USA on recycled paper.

This book is dedicated to every vegan teenager out there. Keep living, keep loving. We're going to change the world, you know.

ACKNOWLEDGMENTS

My wonderful parents, for letting me be vegan in the first place, driving me to meet-ups, buying and cooking vegan food, changing their diets, countless meals and hugs, and being all-around supportive even when they don't understand me.

Bob and Jenna Torres for encouraging, supporting, and making this project possible, as well as for always providing inspiration, energy, and peace of mind through their vegan media empire (and for introducing me to the Dead Kennedys).

Every member of VegKC and some of the finest vegans in all Portlandia for support, activism, friendship, and lots of really great food.

Vegan teens everywhere for inspiring me to write this book. As cheesy as it sounds, we are the future of the movement, so let's make it a good one.

Exceptional humans in Oregon, Kansas, Utah, Colorado, and beyond for believing in me ferociously, filling my day-to-days with happiness, and being my people.

CONTENTS

★

Part Three: Food

Part Four: Now Stay Vegan!

PREFACE TO THE SECOND EDITION

Wow. That's all I can say right now, wow. When I started writing this book, I was a starry-eyed sixteen-year-old who lived in Kansas and had been vegan for only a few months. Today, I'm twenty and halfway done with college in the most vegan-friendly city in the nation. I wrote this book to help other vegan teenagers figure out how to do their vegan thang as happily as possible, yes, but I also wrote it because I wanted immediately to get my hands dirty, to be part of this movement that transformed the way I thought in a lasting and positive way. I didn't give a crap that I was in high school, I wanted something and I did it anyway. I hope that being vegan gives you some of that same fire. Dealing with unsupportive parents and asinine classmates can be frustrating, but trust me—you are on the right track. If you want to live your life as a big "screw you" to injustice and apathy, as a celebration of delicious food and health and awesome people doing awesome things, you are on the right track. Through this book and through being vegan I've met some of the coolest people and had some of the most awesome opportunities of my life. Believe me when I tell you that you can have the same experience.

That said, after several years my perspective has widened. Especially when you're a new vegan, it's easy to think that your experience of veganism now will be your experience of veganism forever, and that's often not the case. Like everything, veganism is a process of growth and it changes alongside you. Wherever you are—whether you're just kinda-maybe-thinking about going vegan, whether you've been vegan for years and years, whether you dabbled in it for a while and want to see if you can do more than dabble now—I hope that this book gives you a sense of peace and purpose. It may seem complicated and hard to others, but that's really all being vegan is—a vision of a peaceful world, and a drive to make that vision a reality, no matter how young or isolated or unsure you might be.

Introduction

Maybe you just went vegan. Maybe you're contemplating going vegan, but are wondering a few things, like...what do vegans eat, especially teenage vegans who are still living at home and may lack cooking skill? What do you tell your parents if they're against you being vegan? How do you deal with non-vegan friends who just don't get it? How do you stay healthy as a vegan? Why *should* you be vegan, anyway?

When I went vegan, I didn't know anybody else who was vegan, much less a vegan my age who was wise with all the ways of the vegan world. This created a lot of feelings, first of all, loneliness. The very beginning of your veganism, I think, tends to be the loneliest if you don't have a vegan mentor-type person. Suddenly, just about everything is new and different, and it can be tough if you have no one in your life who knows how that feels. Being vegan as a teenager is drastically different than being a vegan adult, so even if you have vegan friends older than you, it's slightly alienating. You're a little set away from adult vegans because you're a teenager; you're a little set away from other teenagers because you're vegan.

Well, my hope is that this book brings you closer to both sets. *Generation V* is for all the teenagers out there who wander around just-adding-water to boxes of vegan food, trying their hardest to defend their choices to their friends, and thinking they're the only vegan teenager in the world. Things can be *so* much better! Read this and go forth spreading the vegan love, filled with knowledge and yummy food like the crazy vegan you are.

Love, Claire

My Vegan Story

★

The process of going vegan is like the experience of being vegan: although there may be a lot of common ground, it really is unique to every person. I don't mean that "vegan" by definition means different things to different people but that everyone's experience of going vegan and how veganism fits into the rest of their life is different. It's easy to see going vegan as the end of a journey, but for me, it was a prologue to another journey that I hope will never be over.

In June 2005, at the tender age of fourteen, I was talking to a friend of mine. Nicole was a vegetarian, and, although we had been friends for some time, I didn't know this. It came up casually, and we didn't really talk about it in detail. But since she was the first vegetarian I'd met, I became curious as to why anyone would have problems with eating meat. I have a habit of researching every part of something I get interested in, and this was no different. I went online, determined to find out why ethical vegetarians are ethical vegetarians. I read a thing or two. I watched a thing or two. I started suspecting that vegetarians might actually have good reasons for passing up meat. Before I could really get started, though, my mom called me for lunch. It was chicken. I ate it slowly, with a sneaking suspicion that this would be the last meat I would eat. I didn't like looking at it and had no idea how I would tell my parents I wanted to be vegetarian, so instead of eating something else, I just read while I ate, picking around the meat. When

I was done, I went back to researching, and the more I found out, the more I was convinced that there was no possible way I could continue eating meat. Then I watched Goldfinger's music video for their song "Free Me," and that was it. It hit me: meat is dead. Meat used to be part of a living body, and now it's on my plate, and I support that with my money. I became a vegetarian.

When I had gotten used to my new status as a vegetarian, I started thinking about how I would break the news to my mom. After some thought I figured the best way would be only ask her if I could try out vegetarianism, temporarily. This would probably freak her out less than announcing that I wanted to be vegetarian for as long as I could, and less freaked out would mean more open.

So I tried this, and it worked. I tried to be casual about it, and didn't get specific about the things I had found out, only how they made me feel. My mom wanted to know where I would get protein and was a little reluctant at first, but in the end she was okay with it. (My dad was okay with it, too, but he's okay with just about anything.)

Time went on, and I loved being vegetarian. It was a million times easier than I thought it would be, and, since I knew the truth about meat, I had absolutely no desire for it (and meat analogues were delicious anyway).

I knew what vegan meant, but I thought it was too extreme and didn't know why some people chose to avoid all animal products rather than just meat. I thought that vegans were just paranoid vegetarians who weren't big fans of food. Like a lot of lacto-ovo vegetarians, I believed that dairy and eggs could be taken from cows and chickens without harming them. At the time, I thought that meat was the only unethical animal product and that, because dairy and eggs weren't dead animal parts, they didn't involve harming animals at all. I never once thought about what would happen to laying hens and dairy cows after they laid their eggs or were milked. Looking back from where I am now, it seems impossible to me that I could ever think that animal agriculture could encompass both the horrors of meat production and my ideal of cruelty-free eggs and dairy. The only thing that makes sense is that either all factory-farmed animals are treated humanely or they're all treated with cruelty, but back then, I believed that utter cruelty and acceptable, humane treatment existed within the same system.

Things changed for me in about August of that year. While looking at something about vegetarianism to show my mom (who was still easing out of her reluctance), I stumbled across information about how dairy cows and laying hens are really treated for the first time. I was convinced that vegetarianism was enough, though, and basically ignored what I read and saw, simply thinking, "That's too bad, but I'm already a vegetarian," with a shrug. I couldn't repress what I had found out for long, and a few days later I casually mentioned to my mom that I might like to be vegan. She shook her head, saying she thought it would be too drastic, and I forgot about the idea—for a while, at least.

The more I thought about veganism and the reasons I was a vegetarian in the first place, the more I realized that being only a vegetarian wasn't being true to my beliefs. I didn't think that animals belonged to humans or that they should suffer for something as stupid and unnecessary as a cheeseburger. I dreamed of a world where all animals were thought of in about the same way as dogs and cats—different from humans, definitely, but still beings with their own interests in being alive and well. Companions, fellow earthlings—not property or machines. And yet, I came to realize, I was going back on these beliefs every time I ate eggs or dairy.

This bothered me, but because my mom didn't accept it, I didn't go vegan—entirely, that is. I didn't like the taste of milk and had been drinking soymilk since before I was even vegetarian (simply because chocolate soymilk is delicious) and I stopped really eating eggs or dairy, at least by themselves. I would eat them if they were hidden in something, and I didn't yet know that things

7

like whey or glycerin were animal-derived. I figured that this added up to me being a near-vegan and that cutting out the teeny tiny bits of animal product left in my diet would do so little for the animals that it wasn't worth bothering about or worrying my parents.

Now it was October 2005. I started to realize that, yes, it's possible to make baked goods (and all the other non-vegan foods I was worried I would miss) without eggs and dairy, and, yes, tiny amounts of animal products do add up. I was really worried that my parents won't be cool with my veganism, though, so I started to be a secret oh-so-close-to-vegan. My thinking was that, if my parents didn't know I was purposely avoiding the granola bars in our house that listed whey as the only non-vegan ingredient, for example, they wouldn't make me eat them, and that if they knew I was purposely avoiding them and would like a vegan kind of granola bar, they would get all "Veganism is bad! Stop!" and make me eat even less-vegan things.

So a secret near-vegan I was. Occasionally I would eat tiny amounts of animal products, but this was only because my parents didn't know that I still wanted to be vegan and therefore the only vegan food they bought me was vegan on accident. A few weeks went by, and I decided that it would be my New Year's resolution to go vegan. All the way, zero animal products, parents fully aware, the whole shebang on January first. I figured this would give me plenty of time to get my parents used to the idea.

Starting in November, I decided I would eat vegan in bursts of a few days to see what it was really like. With two months of casually getting my mom to accept the idea of her daughter being a vegan and two months of practicing being a real vegan for days at a time, I figured by January I'd be golden. During one of the first of these vegan trial periods, in early November, I was at the grocery with my mom. She wanted to know if I wanted to try a different kind of granola bar, handing me the package. I pretended to be fascinated with the back of the box, while really checking the ingredients list to see if they were vegan. They weren't, so I simply said, "Nah." "Why?" my mom asked. "They look good."

At that moment, I realized I had to be vegan. I don't know what it was about that moment—snack foods rarely inspire deep shifts in my moral fiber—but I just had to. Everything came together for me. I knew that vegetarianism was truly not in line with my ethics. I knew that going vegan wouldn't be limiting the variety or flavor of my diet in any way. I knew that being vegan was just as healthy, if not more so, as being a vegetarian or a meat-eater. I just knew I had to, could, needed to be vegan. My mom had to know, and if she didn't like it... tough. She was apprehensive about my vegetarianism at first and now she was so supportive, so would veganism really be that different?

"Because they've got whey, and whey is from milk, and...I want to be vegan." She sighed, but I continued, gently, telling her I'd been trying it at home, pointing out all the vegan food that was around us there in the store, and, just like when I went vegetarian, suggesting that I merely try it out even though I was past that and now serious about it. She gave in to my vegan wiles.

I was giddy! I was finally going to be a real live *vegan!* I had a whirlwind of different feelings: pride—I'd finally done it!; joy—no more animal suffering in my life!; but also loneliness—at the time I was the only vegan I knew; and confusion—what do I really *do?* Gradually, I met vegans, read books about veganism, learned to cook, and here I sit, a very happy and healthy young vegan writing a book. Life's pretty good.

As I said, veganism has been a journey in itself for me. As I have matured as a person, so have my motivations for being vegan. It used to be that I was simply against the treatment of sentient beings in factory farms. Factory farms were gross and made me sad. While factory farms haven't changed and neither has the ability of animals to feel pain and fear, my primary reason for being an herbivore now is more political—I don't think sentient beings should be treated as commodities. Even on the nicest, most humane farm in the world, beings with their own interests are treated as if they're simply there to serve humans, and they're not. They're not humans, but they're not humans and they're not objects, and no matter how nicely you treat them you still enforce that they belong to us and it's okay to eat them as long as we do it nicely. Depriving others of their autonomy because of a prejudice is the same source as racism and sexism—more on this later.

So, all you non-vegans out there, I bet you're wondering what it was really like to go vegan. Difficult? Nope, it's only as difficult as you make it for yourself. Here's the thing: you have reason for wanting to be vegan, right? You do. If you find out about how animals are treated in factory farms, and think it's too bad, but still want to eat animals—that's not going vegan. I mean, that's great to at least be thinking about it, but it's very different from actually making the decision to boycott all animal products in your life. If you make that decision, it's not like you're dying to eat a big plate of scrambled eggs and be "normal." Your knowledge of how that plate of eggs came about overpowers any desire you have to be the same as most people, to eat anything off the menu from any restaurant, etc. because you know and feel that it's *wrong*. Plus, eggs are chicken menstruation and that's just creepy. After a while, you just stop seeing animal products as food...or as the norm.

If you're not vegan, let me try and get you to feel what it's like for us vegans. Imagine there's something you've been doing your entire life. It's fun, convenient, and you're used to it. Why would you do anything else? Because, you find out, every time you do that thing, horrible things happen. Things that are horrible in themselves but also speak of a larger worldview that doesn't sit well with you, that you wouldn't dream of if you were queen or king of the universe. Naturally, you stop doing whatever it was you were doing, and you feel a lot better. It's not that hard, and you even wonder why you didn't stop sooner.

But, here's the thing: Everybody else still does that thing. You know, deep down, that if they truly knew what was going on and what their actions meant, most of them would stop in a heartbeat, but nobody knows. When they're exposed to even a hint of the truth, they become defensive, shrug it off, make jokes, and give excuses. You wonder why they have such a skewed vision of the way you now live and why they're like you in some ways but very different in others. Dealing with other people can be frustrating, but when they're receptive and respond well, it's wonderful, so it all balances out. Sometimes you are livid at the world for being the way it is, sometimes you're elated because you know on some basic level that things *will* change, have to change, and you love being part of that change. Sometimes you feel like you're the only human on the planet that cares about anything, sometimes you feel profoundly and invisibly connected to all the other people that do. Sometimes you feel that all your attempts at changing things amount to nothing, sometimes you think that even the small things do a world of good.

So, that's what it feels like. Is it easy? Not always. Is it tons of fun? Sometimes. Is it worth it? Oh yeah!

ALL THE COOL KIDS
ARE ETHICAL VEGANS

★

If someone refused to believe that women can do the same things men can and thought their only purpose was to serve men, you would probably be horrified and call that sexism in an instant. It doesn't matter if a person espouses their sexism in very obvious ways, like abusing their wife or denying a woman a job purely on the basis of her sex, or very subtle ones, like throwing the word *slut* around nonstop. Either way, you would recognize that it's preferring males to females simply because they lack a Y chromosome, and that it's wrong. It's believing that all women—no matter how intelligent, creative, or strong they may be—are inferior to men for no other reason than that they are women, and that's unfair. I don't doubt that you're against sexism, even if you're not a diligent reader of Feministing.com and you've never heard the name Judith Butler. You don't have to be very familiar with feminist theory to recognize sexism as an unethical ideology, because you can easily understand that it's unjust to hold something like sex as the only marker for a human's worth. Sex is arbitrary, that is, not chosen, so it is unfair to use it to judge worth. This simple principle leads you to see that women do not deserve to be regulated solely to the roles of wife, mother, and homemaker. You also don't need a degree in gender studies to find examples of sexism throughout history—that women had to struggle for many years to earn the right to vote, for one example. It just seems to you like common ethical knowledge that sexism is an unjust system of thought.

If someone told you that people of color couldn't have intellectual thought on the same level as white people, that would be clear-cut racism and you'd be appalled. That person could be as boldly racist as to support reestablishing slavery, or they could simply not want to be friends with a Hispanic person for no other reason than that she is Hispanic. In either case, that person would believe that people who are not their race are inferior, for no other reason than their skin is a different color, even if the other person is actually superior to them in some way (say, more intelligent). You would be able to see without difficulty that skin color or ethnicity is no reason to oppress someone. You would also be able to clearly understand, without having spent time reading volumes on race and racism, that it's unjust to mistreat people or force them to serve you merely because they are of a different race (or at all, but that's a different story). The fact that racism is wrong is very easily understood and believed by anyone who wishes to be called ethical in today's society. Race is an arbitrary characteristic, so we simply don't use it to determine a person's worth.

Throughout history, instances of widespread sexism and racism are common. Let's look at the slave trade for one example. At one time, almost all Westerners saw it as a legitimate economic industry. It was convenient and the socially accepted norm. Nobody really saw the way their person-turned-"product" got to them. Now, though, we see the slave trade as an atrocity. It's not that people hundreds of years ago were savages; it's just that it took a few dedicated and forward-thinking individuals to seriously examine what was going on, realize it was immoral, and to change the minds of the masses.

At this point, you might be wondering what the heck all this has to do with veganism. Well, what if someone thought that nonhuman animals were simply incapable of feeling pain, joy, sorrow, or loss?* What if they thought that animals have no interests of their own and are only here to serve humans? That, my friend, would be speciesism. *Speciesism* is the word for oppressing those not of your species and using them for your species's benefit, just like sexism is oppressing those not of your sex and using them for your sex's benefit, and just like racism is oppressing those not of your race and using them for your race's benefit. It might be your knee-jerk reaction to be appalled that anyone would compare speciesism to sexism or racism, but this is simple moral logic and comparison. You don't have to believe that the plight of one chicken is as bad as the slave trade to recognize speciesism as an unethical ideology that uses arbitrary characteristics to determine worth and value. The comparisons between these three ideologies are numerous.

Today, if you were to mention that you're a vegetarian or vegan, you'll no doubt get at least some people claiming that eating meat, dairy, and eggs is natural, tradition, the way things have always been. You'll probably hear that that's what animals are for and get asked why else they would be here, what purpose would they serve.

If you were to travel back in time and talk to a slave owner or an opponent of women's suffrage, you would hear those *exact* arguments. At certain points in time, most men thought that keeping their wives in the kitchen and nursery was simply what women were for. They thought that letting women hold a job outside the home and being successful at it defied tradition and "how things are supposed to be." Most white people thought that African Americans and other races were "meant" to be enslaved and had no other purpose but to serve whites. Now, right now, the majority of humans—humans who would call themselves ethical, rational, good people—don't even consider that

---

*Go give your dog lots of love and attention and see how she reacts. Then take away her food, punch her around, and see how she reacts, and then tell me you still think animals are emotionless automatons. (Note: I do not support the actual punching around of anyone's dog.)

exploiting animals is a matter of ethics, just something that we've always done. I'm sure people believe in some way that animals have interests in being alive, happy, keeping their babies, and being free from pain, but few people act on these beliefs. When they ask what other purpose animals would serve, they assume that animals *must* have some human purpose to serve, that their existence is only justified by having some human purpose to *need* to serve. Indeed, almost all Westerners see the production of meat, dairy, and eggs as legitimate economic industries. It is convenient and the socially accepted norm. Nobody really sees the way their animals-turned-"products" get to them, though the way it gets to them is atrocious...does this sound familiar?

Some people are probably going to tell you that animals are not as intelligent as humans, and that's why our treatment of them is ethically justified. But you really can't defend using someone's mental inferiority to you as a basis for abusing them. A newborn couldn't communicate with you in the same language you use, but that's no reason to subject her to pain or treat her as an object because it's convenient for you. Somebody would probably say that a baby could and will learn language, and animals can't, but think of gorillas and other primates who have learned to use human sign language. Many other animals could probably be taught to communicate in the same way humans do, but why do we humans have the intrinsic ability to judge what constitutes communication? Other animals communicate with members of their species perfectly— if they couldn't, they wouldn't survive. We haven't really learned to communicate with animals using their "languages," and we're not stupid, but just because animals do not communicate using human language, they're stupid. What kind of logic is that? People also assume that pigs, chickens, and cows are stupid even though they have interacted with animals like cats and dogs and have seen that those animals are definitely not stupid.

If these ideas are new to you, they might still seem strange. Maybe they make sense to you in your head, but you don't yet see how they play out every day in the world or what they have to do with your life. Let's examine just how we turn thinking, feeling beings into commodities.

The first and most obvious transformation of animals into products is turning animals into food. This section will serve as a primer for learning about this, exploring the different ways that different animals are used for different foods. This section's main sources are books rather than websites, which can be seen as more biased and/or exaggerated than books. This is not to say that the internet does not have legitimate information about factory farms but to leave as little room as possible for skeptics to deny the treatment of animals, as many will when you give them something from, say, a PETA website. One book this section relies on heavily is *Meat Market: Animals, Ethics, and Money* by Erik Marcus (Brio Press, 2005). Marcus's book is sourced from respected agricultural journals, and rather than wanting you to go, "Aww," and see factory-farmers as heartless sadists, Marcus gives the industry's economic explanation for the extreme confinement, neglect, and abuse seen in factory farms. If you doubt or want further information on anything covered in this next section, I highly encourage you to read Marcus's book. Another book this section uses is *Slaughterhouse: The Shocking Story of Greed, Neglect, and Inhumane Treatment Inside the U.S. Meat Industry* by Gail A. Eisnitz (Prometheus Books, 1997). A great deal of the information in *Slaughterhouse* is thanks to the countless hours Eisnitz spent interviewing real, live factory-farm workers about their jobs, and I would also highly recommend reading the book if you want further information.

The United States has raised and subsequently killed more than ten billion (that's billion with a b, and that's a number greater than that of humans in the world) animals per year for animal agriculture since 2003 (Marcus). Math is fun—ten billion animals per year is about 833,333,333 animals a month, 192,307,692 animals a week, and 27,397,260 animals a day. That's 1,141,552 animals an hour. In the time it takes you to read this sentence, hundreds of animals will have their lives ended to become someone's meal. And remember, these staggering figures are in the United States alone.

With such a demand for animal products, factory farms can gain or lose great sums of money due to the smallest differences between them and their competitors. "Between 1950 and 2001, the cost of the average new house surged...nearly 1500 percent. Over the same period, new car prices climbed more than 1400 percent...the price of animal products has lagged far behind the overall inflation rate. The price of milk is up only about 350 percent between 1950 and 2003. And, during that time, the prices of eggs and chicken meat haven't even doubled" (ibid., 7) The comparatively small changes in price for animal products show what a competitive market the animal agriculture industry is. Not having to spend an extra penny or getting another penny's worth of profit from something translates to enormous variations in revenue. Marcus explains that this principle is the driving force behind the treatment of animals in modern agriculture. If it's profitable to fit as many chickens (which are cheap) as possible into as few cages (which are costly) as possible, a factory farm is not going to put itself into debt because it may be a little sad that the chickens are so crowded. It's as simple as that. Similarly, if an egg-laying outfit can hike up the prices on its eggs, due to their being advertised as free-range, while enacting as few changes in actual treatment as possible, it's going to do that, too. People in charge of factory farms don't overcrowd/neglect animals for the sheer fun of it; they do so for the sheer fun of making money. Understanding this is key to understanding why animals are treated the way they are. There is scarcely an aspect of factory farming that isn't because of money.

Egg-laying hens

Once laying chicks are hatched, they are separated by sex. Female chicks will go on to lay eggs in cramped cages like their mothers. Male chicks do not lay eggs and, since they are the children of hens bred to lay large numbers of eggs rather than gain large amounts of weight, grow too slowly to be raised for meat. The male chicks, being useless to animal agriculture, are killed. Gassing is one method, but the more common one is maceration—in other words, death by being ground alive. Sometimes male chicks are simply thrown out with the trash, where they die from smothering and lack of air. Over 272 million male chicks were killed in America in 2002. (Marcus, 16)

The remaining females must then have their beaks seared. Since they will spend their lives surrounded by so many other hens in such tight space, it is very common for the hens to begin to literally go crazy from stress and confinement and to peck the hens around them. (Imagine living in a closet with five strangers for most of your life.) To ensure that the hens do not peck each other to death, egg-laying facilities sear off portions of the hens' beaks. The industry refers to this as "beak trimming," but beak trimming sounds like it hurts about as much as clipping your toenails. Think instead of having a part of your mouth removed with a hot blade with no help of anesthesia, because this is exactly what happens. A worker picks up a chick and places her in a device that slices off a portion of her beak. Chicks suffer pain from this procedure for as long as five or six weeks after it is performed. Accidents are common, and many chicks die of hunger or thirst when too great a portion of their beak is removed, and it becomes painful to eat and drink.

After seventeen weeks of life (keep in mind that around a third of this time may be spent in pain from beak-searing), the chicks are taken from the hatchery to an egg-laying facility. There, they spend their lives with eight or more other hens inside one battery cage. A battery cage is the industry's standard space for hens. It is made of wire mesh and is about fifty-nine inches square, roughly the size of a filing cabinet drawer. With so many hens in one of these, each hen has the living space about the same size as a sheet of ordinary notebook paper—not a whole lot larger than the book you have in your hands. Urine and feces from the hens inside the battery cages fall on other hens in cages below. When a hen gets a limb or her head stuck in the wire, she will often die of starvation or dehydration due to being unable to free herself and reach food and water. Even if she does not get caught between the wire, she may die of starvation/dehydration anyway— she has her feet wrapped around wire all day every day and soon she can no longer move her feet to get to food and water. She and her cagemates will frequently rub their feathers away and rub their skin raw from being pressed up against the wire twenty-four hours a day.

An egg-laying hen lives in this way for around two years. It takes over twenty-four hours of this suffering for a hen to produce just one egg. In nature, hens can live to be up to eleven years old and lay between fifty and a hundred eggs per year. Laying eggs at such an unnatural rate takes severe tolls on the hen's body. If you're a girl, think about having a period every three days instead of every month and think of how your body would feel. Just as you would suffer extreme anemia in such a situation, hens that lay eggs so often suffer from extreme osteoporosis due to all the calcium they lose to make eggshells. Their bones are frail and often break (and go untreated). After a while, a hen's body gives up and the rate at which she lays eggs plummets. She will be deprived of food for up to two weeks at a time (the industry calls this "forced molting") in order to raise her laying rates. The process of forced molting can continue for up to six month's of a hen's life, causing death in some birds and severe weight loss in others.

At between two and three years old, an egg-laying hen is slaughtered. Her meat is used for pet food, feed for other factory-farmed animals, and some human food.

"Broiler" chickens (and other poultry)

All poultry are treated basically the same, so I will focus on chickens raised for meat, as they are the most common. The animal agriculture industry refers to chickens being raised for meat as "broilers." These chickens live in concrete-floored warehouses, receiving less than one square foot of living space per chicken. Most broiler houses hold at least twenty thousand chickens at once.

At seven weeks old, these chickens get to see the sky and breathe fresh air for the first time as they are loaded onto trucks to go to the slaughterhouse. Since there is no time for them to convert any more food into profit (meat), they are no longer fed. Many birds die en route to the slaughterhouse, mostly due to the extreme weather conditions they sometimes face.

Workers take the chickens from the transport trucks and shackle them, upside-down. The next step in the killing process is an electrified bath for the chickens. While slaughterhouses maintain that this is for a humane killing, the birds usually only get their heads dipped in the water, rendering them immobile rather than unconscious. As they are motionless, a blade slits each bird's throat. Most birds regain movement after this and can feel the pain of a slit throat in a very real way. "It unfortunately makes good economic sense to keep stunning amperage to minimal levels. Stunning a bird with sufficient current to cause cardiac arrest often causes convulsions strong enough to break bones. These broken bones will downgrade carcasses, resulting in the slaughterhouse receiving less money per bird" (Marcus, 25) The chickens usually bleed to death and are plucked and processed mechanically.

Chicken slaughterhouses kill at a rate of about two chickens per second. This is many times faster than any other slaughterhouse. This is largely because chickens are so much smaller than other animals killed for food. It takes many more chickens to equal the amount of meat provided by one pig, and still more to equal the meat from one cow. In 2000, more than eight billion chickens were killed for meat in the U.S. Remember that the most recent figure for the *total* number of animals killed in America is ten billion.

Dairy cows and veal calves

Dairy cows are raised in two kinds of facilities. The first is a fenced outdoor lot. Cows are kept in this crowded pen, standing and lying in their own excrement (how would it be economically beneficial to clean?) and eating from troughs on the pen's perimeter. The second kind of facility is a metal-roofed shed where cows are kept chained in individual stalls and are fed by conveyor belt. Dairy cows are kept pregnant for nine months out of every year and produce over 2,000 gallons of milk yearly. This brutal cycle of continuous pregnancy and unnatural milk production leads to severe stress on the cows' bodies, often resulting in disease, lameness, and other health problems.

Cows are artificially inseminated at least once a year. After a calf is born, the mother does not produce regular milk immediately. Instead, she gives a substance called colostrum, which has a distinct flavor and cannot be sold as normal milk. Nearly 9 percent of calves die before their mothers start producing regular milk, about two days after the cows give birth. However, once colostrum production ends, mother and child are separated. The cow is led off to a milking parlor as her calf is taken away to another part of the dairy. Once she returns, she finds her calf missing and will often hysterically bellow for days as she attempts to locate her child.

Now, the cow will spend her days alternating between her stall or the lot and the milking parlor. Because of such stress on the udders, many cows—about one in five—develop a condition called mastitis. When cows have mastitis, their udders swell painfully and produce pus to combat the infection (our bodies do that, too).

When her milk production begins to wane, a cow will be impregnated again. A cow usually has three babies in her life. Her female calves will grow up to be dairy cows. Her male calves, on the other hand, will become veal. It's a common vegan saying that every glass of milk contains a small hunk of veal, and while this is not literally true, every glass of milk comes from the mother of a veal calf. Thus, if you support the dairy industry, you support the veal industry. Period.

I'm sure you know about the horrendous treatment veal calves receive. They are auctioned off when "still slick from the womb" (Marcus, 38) and deliberately fed to be anemic. They spend their very short lives in tiny crates and this, in combination with the inadequate nutrition they receive, results in very soft flesh sought after by many gourmands.

Beef cattle

Unlike most other animals, calves raised for beef have a pretty good life up to a point. Since breeding for beef cattle is so different than breeding for chickens, dairy cows, or pigs, they're born with relatively normal bodies and miss out on a lot of the health problems that other animals have due to their unnatural growth. For the first six to eight months of the calf's life, he actually gets to graze on open pasture with his mother. Grazing land is subsidized by the U.S. government, so it's extremely cheap to pay for a calf's open living space.

After these six or so months, the rancher comes to take the calf. The calf's mother usually has a hood thrown over her head, so she won't see her child being taken away and hurt the rancher. Once the calf is taken away, he is branded, dehorned, and castrated, all without the use of anesthesia. Then he is loaded onto a truck or train and taken to the feedlot.

During the four or five months young cattle spend at a feedlot, they will often gain four hundred to five hundred pounds. Although cattle are used to eating grasses, they are fed corn at feedlots because that makes them gain weight faster. They often take liver damage and other health problems due to this unnatural feed. Feeding corn to cows also messes with the pH of their digestive system, so feedlot operations will usually load their corn with antibiotics to combat the bacteria growing in the cows' digestive systems. A calf's life at a feedlot consists of eating this corn and standing around with thousands of other steers on a floor of dirt and their own manure.

When they have reached a sufficient weight, steers are then transported to the slaughterhouse. These rides often last more than sixteen hours at a time, and are so crowded that if a steer falls, he faces a great risk of being trampled to death by his fellows. After this ride, a steer lives in a corral until it is his turn for the killing floor.

Prior to the Humane Slaughter Act of 1978, steers simply had their throats slit. Now, they are killed with a captive bolt pistol. This pistol sends a steel rod between the steer's eyes, with the intention of inducing a coma so he is unconscious while he is butchered. However, these captive bolt pistols are prone to failure, and the great speed of the killing line does not ensure that there is enough time per cow to for a surefire coma. Often, the bolt will indeed go through a steer's skull, but not hit the exact spot on the brain needed to knock the cow unconscious. Thus, many steers continue through the killing fully conscious, still in pain from just receiving a bolt to the brain. Marcus explains this, referencing an article by the Washington Post about slaughterhouses ("They Die Piece by Piece"). When bolt guns misfire, "fully conscious animals have been sent down the line. The most disturbing part of the Post's revelations pertained to the cattle who remained conscious even as they were being butchered. One slaughterhouse worker interviewed by the Post said he saw conscious cattle make it all the way to the disemboweling machine."

American slaughterhouses kill one steer every nine seconds, just enough time to shoot the steer, not to check to see if he has been shot accurately. Workers who slow the line to check or to reshoot an animal will most likely lose their job to someone who doesn't slow down the profit by slowing the line, so workers simply do not slow the line even if they know a steer is still conscious. The same article by the *Washington Post* details this, saying, "An effective stunning requires a precision shot, which workers must deliver hundreds of times daily to balky, frightened animals [who] frequently weigh 1,000 pounds or more. Within 12 seconds of entering the chamber, the fallen steer is shackled to a moving chain to be bled and butchered by other workers in a fast-moving production line."

Pigs

After female pigs chosen to become breeder sows reach eight months of age, they are impregnated for the first time, beginning a grueling cycle similar to that endured by dairy cows. Sows spend the rest of their lives either pregnant or nursing and are impregnated every four to five months. To fit more sows in a smaller space, pregnant sows are kept in what are called gestation crates. These metal crates are similar to the crates that veal calves live in. A sow stays in her crate for her entire pregnancy, around four months. A few days before she gives birth, she is moved into a "farrowing crate," which is very similar to a gestation crate, but with lower-level pockets for piglets. Eisnitz interviewed a worker at a pig factory farm about this move. "'[The workers] beat the shit out of [the pigs] to get them inside the crates because they don't want to go. This is their only chance to walk around, get a little exercise, and they don't want to go,' a worker said. Another employee at a different farm described the routine use of gate rods used to the beat the sows bloody. 'One guy smashed a sow's nose in so bad that she ended up dying of starvation'" (Eisnitz, 219).

Since they spend virtually all of their lives in tight crates, deprived of virtually any sensory simulation, sows suffer mentally. Sows will often develop psychological trauma,

Marcus says, due to "the emotional toll connected to confinement. The boredom resulting from isolation can give rise to an abnormal psychological state called stereotypy, in which sows do the same senseless repetitive motion thousands of times each day. Sows have also been witnessed trying to attack the crates that keep them so tightly confined." (Marcus, 30)

Piglets nurse for around seventeen days in confinement (compared with around three months in nature). During this time, more than 5 percent of piglets are crushed while nursing, and around 3 percent die from starvation or diarrhea. Once the remaining piglets are weaned, they undergo castration, tail-docking, and ear-notching, all without anesthesia. Pork from uncastrated males has a distinct and unpleasant odor. The overcrowding in factory farms leads pigs to bite each other's tails out of anger. Cutting off portions of the tail is cheaper than providing adequate space. Ear-notching means that deep scores are cut into piglet's ears for identification purposes. While their fellows undergo these processes, piglets are housed in battery cages similar to those laying hens live in.

Tiny piglets would be certainly crushed to death if they were taken from their mothers' sides and immediately put with adult pigs about to be slaughtered. So, the piglets spend several weeks in what the industry calls "nurseries." These are usually large sheds with wooden or concrete flooring. Here, the piglets are moved from their mothers' milk to solid food. Often, this "food" is dried blood plasma taken from other slaughterhouses— it's cheap and it makes pigs grow, and that means profit. After they have gone from around ten to around forty pounds, they are then placed with other adult pigs in "finishing sheds."

At finishing sheds, the pigs gain about six times their original weight. Most sheds house up to a thousand pigs. Of these, only around 10 percent ever go outside. The rest spend 100 percent of their time inside in crowded metal pens with concrete, wood, or sometimes earthen floors. These unnatural living surfaces lead to great numbers of joint and foot problems for pigs. The manure pits in these sheds leads to great numbers of lung problems for both pigs and humans alike. The ammonia in pig manure contributes to terrible air quality. Marcus explains, "Studies of lungs taken from slaughtered pigs indicate that between 30 and 70 percent of pigs have developed chronic respiratory disease. Predictably, workers in pig confinement facilities are also at high risk... Researchers have found that at least 25 percent of these workers have respiratory ailments."

Next comes transport to the slaughterhouse. The ride to the slaughterhouse is usually long, and around eighty thousand pigs die each year during it (Marcus, 33). Extreme weather conditions are often endured. Eisnitz interviewed one worker about the results of some of these conditions. "In the wintertime there are always hogs stuck to the sides and floors of the trucks. They go in there with wires or knives and just cut or pry the hogs loose. The skin pulls right off. These hogs were alive when we did this" (Eisnitz, 133).

When they reach the slaughterhouse, pigs are kept in holding pens until it is their turn to die. They are prodded onto a narrow walkway and stunned. Then they have their throats slit and are dunked in the scald tank—a tub of water at 140 degrees Fahrenheit—in order to remove the tiny hairs on their skin. However, as with cows, many pigs remain conscious throughout this process due to the speed of the line. One slaughterhouse worker interviewed by Eisnitz explains this, saying that the numbers of live, conscious animals who make it through the line are "'too many to count. Too many to remember... I've seen hogs [that are supposed to be lying down] on the bleeding conveyor get up after they've been stuck. I've seen hogs in the scalding tub trying to swim.'"

If you, like most people, thought farms were just like the ones in picture books, you're probably reeling. It's shocking how schizophrenic our relationship with animals is. We love animals like dogs and cats, spend our money making sure they're happy and healthy, let them live in our houses and even sleep in our beds, hold them as members of our family, and can see that they can experience a full range of emotions and have distinct personalities. Yet, just for money, just for twenty minutes of a happy mouth, we cage, abuse, and kill other animals who are just as emotional, just as intelligent, just as ready to form relationships with humans, and just as deserving of equality and our respect. Veganism is embracing the idea that all animals, human or non-, have inherent worth and value and should be treated with compassion. Veganism is refusing to believe that some species deserve to be treated wonderfully and some deserve to be treated with cruelty. Veganism is a full and total rejection of the cruelty, the unquestioned ideology, and the schizophrenia of our attitudes towards and treatment of animals. Veganism is denying that sentient beings are commodities, living money, objects that belong to us. Veganism is about equality, compassion, and effecting positive change in the world and yourself. Read on and learn how to be the healthiest, happiest vegan you can be, with the tastiest food, the easiest social life, and the least-annoyed and most-supportive parents.

Part One:
Dealing With...

Chapter One: Parents and Other Family

★

Going vegan as a teen can be more difficult than doing so when you're an adult. Your parents have significantly more control over your life when you're young. You still have to live under their roof, follow their rules (to a certain extent, at least) and depend on them for most, if not all, of your money, clothes, freedom—and food. So, if your parents don't understand/accept/support your decision to cut animal cruelty from your life, it can be very difficult, if not impossible, to be vegan when you're a teenager.

See, when you're an adult—living on your own, paying for everything—veganism's only as hard or easy as you yourself make it. If your parents don't like the idea of you being vegan, it might create a problem at, say, holidays, but won't really impact your day-to-day vegan livin'. If you want to fill your fridge with seitan and soymilk, sport clothes with vegan messages, and spend your time reading books about animal liberation, your parents can't do anything to stop you. If you're a teenager, however, there's a lot your parents can do to stop you. This is where the difficulty comes in.

On the one hand, if they won't let you go vegan and you still really want to, it's too bad because either you wind up eating bad, boring, not-so-nutritious food or being torn up inside as you eat animal products. On the other hand, if your parents make your veganism so difficult that you eventually lose the desire to be vegan, it's too bad because then you're turning your back on your ethics.

But there's a third hand! If you just figure out why your parents are so against the idea of you being vegan and then show them that their misconceptions are just that— misconceptions, that their fears won't come true, and so on. Then you can happily coexist with your non-vegan parents and vice versa! Trust me, it can happen. Maybe your parents envision you morphing into a jaundiced skeleton from a diet of nothing but lentils and green tea. Maybe they're picturing you throwing red paint on fur-wearers and screaming at them at the top of your lungs about animal cruelty. Maybe they think your friends will stop talking to you when you will no longer go to certain fast-food restaurants with them. Whatever the reason(s), use this chapter to help your parents see that you can be vegan and still be a member of your family as happy as you were prevegan.

The rule of thumb for dealing with non-vegan family is: educate yourself thoroughly, and be peaceful and respectful (or as close to it as you can get) when discussing things. Mumbling "I don't know" when they ask you something about veganism or screaming at them about how wrong they are just won't work. Calmly talking about an issue, knowing what you're going to say, and possibly having a few books or articles to back up what you're saying is a much better way of getting your parents (or any other person, really) to see where you're coming from.

Be patient, too. If something doesn't over go over too well one time, bring it up again in a week or two and hope it goes better. Practice what you're going to say beforehand, if you have to. At the very least, even if it keeps going poorly, your parents will see that you're determined.

Some typical parental worries:

"It's just a phase."

This one can be tougher since you can't just calmly show your parents an article or pamphlet, or fill up your brain and then have a discussion with them. *You* have to be the answer, not what you know or what you have read. The best (and sometimes only) way to deal with a parent who is convinced that your veganism is merely a stage you're going through is to stick with it and give it time. Eventually, they will see that you're serious about being vegan.

"You've been brainwashed!"

This is common when you have a vegan friend who showed you the light. A parent will think that you, in your easily impressionable youth, will want to go vegan after this particular persistent friend (who your parents might imagine as a PETA T-shirt–wearing, dreadlock-sporting, pamphlet-flinging punk/hippie combo if they don't know them) did something to make you suddenly want to make a drastic change in your life. For example, when one of my friends wanted to go vegan because of me, her mom's first response was to ask her daughter what "this Claire" had been doing that caused her to want to go veg. Show your parents that you're still your same old self. You just found that veganism makes a lot of ethical (or environmental, nutritional, etc.) sense. If there is a vegan friend whom your parents don't know well and may be apprehensive of, let the friend meet your parents so they can see that he/she is normal and nice and not an angry uber-militant vegan asshole. If they think you've been brainwashed because yesterday you were eating chicken without a care in the world and today you want to throw away all your leather shoes and tested-on-animals body products, tone it down a little, if only to please them. I'm not saying go back to eating animal products so they'll think you're not as "brainwashed," but you have plenty of time to replace your shoes and toiletries and plenty of time to convince your parents that you're serious about this.

"You won't be healthy!"

Ask your parentals why, specifically, they think you won't be healthy on a vegan diet. Do they think you won't get enough calories? Not enough protein, calcium, or iron? That your diet won't be varied enough? Once you find out just why they don't think your body can thrive without animal products, turn to page 59 and show them that, yes, you can be vegan and be just as healthy as you are now, if not more so. Once you do go vegan, if you feel healthier, have more energy, clearer skin, etc. (which happens to a lot of people!) make sure to mention this to your parents, especially if they didn't think you would be healthy. My mom didn't think I would get enough protein at first, but I showed her the facts and changed her mind. I mention all the time how I have more energy during the day and fall asleep easier at night, how I can barely remember the last time I had a stomach ache or cramps, and a bunch of other stuff—now she's the one who'll point out how clear my skin looks since going vegan.

"You'll be teased!"

Parents who think their child will be teased for being vegan are similar to parents who thinks that their child will be teased for sporting knee-high rainbow toe socks or reading on the bus and at every other possible moment (neither of which are bad, and both of which I may or may not have done in my own early youth). When it comes down to it, they're sending their offspring the message to change herself in order to fit in, and that just ain't cool. Tell your parents something to the tune of, "I'm comfortable with who I am, and wanting to be vegan is a part of who I am. I would rather get teased for being confident in being myself than pretend I'm someone else and never get made fun of." It's very hard for a parent to argue with that. It's also good to mention that if your friends were really your friends, they wouldn't tease you, and if they aren't your friends, who really cares what they think?

Parents who are concerned about you being teased also often think not that you'll get teased simply for going vegan, but that in going vegan you automatically become the self-righteous, undernourished, red-paint-flinging pinko commie stereotypical vegan, and *that's* why you'll get teased—or, regardless of whether or not you get teased, they might not want you to become that stereotype at all. This one can be solved best by giving it time. After a while, your parent will see that you're still you, just vegan, and not drastically different.

"You're too old to be sentimental."

In this situation, your parents are trying to enforce the idea that "that's just how it is"—people just eat animal products, that's just the norm, tough luck, kid. They may assume that your desire to be vegan stems from a childlike view of animals as adorable, innocent peers rather than thinking, feeling beings with their own interests and that you're so young that you just don't know how the world works yet. Make sure your parents know that you feel eating animal products is wrong because it forces suffering on a being who experiences sentience, not because it's mean to hurt poor widdle cowsie-wowsies (and chicky-wickies, and I'm done talking like that...). You are between a child and an adult, yes, but try to play up the fact that you're not holding on to your childlike view of animals, but rather that you're getting older and developing the ability to look beyond what's immediately in front of you and live by your ethics.

"Why won't you eat my food?
Don't you love me?"

Let me tell you a story. A few weeks before I went vegan (when I was trying to be a strict vegetarian as much as possible), my mom and I were in the car together and she mentioned the dinner she had made: some kind of chowder that was predominantly milk and cheese. She was so happy about making this lovely vegetarian meal that (she thought) everyone could enjoy together. My mom didn't really know that I was trying to edge my way down the path to veganism, and I wasn't about to tell her since I thought that she would make me eat more animal products than I would eat if she didn't know. So I asked her if I could have something else for dinner, and she wanted to know why. I tried to avoid it, mumbling "because," but she kept at it, and eventually I told her that I wanted to be vegan and why. She sighed and said something like "But I made it and I thought you would like it...it's vegetarian...I thought we could all eat it together." I did end up eating something more plant-based that night, but what I'm trying to get at is that some parents can take it as a blow to them personally when you reject their food. I'm not saying you should eat a ham-and-cheese omelette if it would make your dad happy, but that a lot of parents forget that you're only turning down what they make you because it contains animal products. My mom made that chowder with the best of intentions, thinking I would be happy because it's vegetarian, only to see me turn up my nose at it.

In this situation, explain to your parents that it's not the fact that they made it that's causing you to refuse the food, just that it's not vegan. Stress that you're not trying to be difficult and you're not rejecting their food for rejection's sake, but that this is something important to you now. You probably have a food or foods that you've never liked, and maybe your parents have avoided cooking that food in the past for you. Bring this up and mention how veganism isn't really that different. When they do take the time and effort to cook you something vegan, be sure to thank and praise them for it. They'll remember that you liked it and might do it again!

Personally, I have never appreciated my mother's cooking more than now that I'm vegan. When I would eat whatever, I thought she made me food simply because I had to eat. Now that I'm vegan, every time she makes me something special, I really know it's because she cares about me and my well-being. When we go visit my extended family and I live in vegan hell (oh, okay, vegan limbo) for a few days, my mom always helps me to make sure I have plenty of delicious and nutritious things to eat, and every time this happens, I appreciate my mother so much more than I did when I was an omnivore.

"I'm not cooking anything special."

Translation #1: I don't know *how* to cook anything special. Most parents (and people in general, really) who aren't familiar with vegan food will assume it's salad, plain tofu, lentils, the neighbor's shrubs, etc. If your parents believe that vegan cooking will be difficult and require a thousand trips to a thousand different health food stores, they most likely won't want to learn about it, especially if you're unwilling to help. If you show that you're willing to learn how to cook and to organize some kind of schedule—maybe your parents will cook something for you every other day, and the rest of the time you'll cook for yourself—they might soften up and grab a cookbook or two (see Chapter 5 for a list of some great vegan cookbooks).

This, for example, is how things worked out in my family. At first, my mom didn't want to cook anything special for me, and I didn't know how to cook, so I basically lived on mixes and frozen meals for the first month or two of my veganism. Then she found a recipe that she veganized for me, and then I found cookbooks. Gradually, we both learned how to cook yummy vegan meals and loved it. Right now, we don't have any sort of "Claire makes dinner on these nights" kind of thing, but it ends up being about half-and-half. I cook dinner three or four nights of the week and my parents do the rest, and, usually, we all eat the same vegan dinner together—I was lucky that I went vegan after my brothers left for college. Your parents might be in a tough spot if you're vegan but have non-vegan siblings—a lot of parents (including mine) assume that since the vegan kid isn't happy with an omnivorous meal, the non-vegan kid(s) won't be happy with a vegan meal. However, this isn't true—delicious food is delicious food and the fact that the food is cruelty-free doesn't make it any less so! Maybe your younger siblings are young enough that they like to do whatever you're doing and would love the idea of eating something special that you want the family to eat. Maybe your older siblings are old enough that they've come across different kinds of ethnic foods and know that they're delicious. It may be a good idea to point out to your parents that your family has eaten a lot of vegan (or easily veganized) food at dinner before—think stir-fries, spaghetti with meatless marinara, vegetable soup, bean burritos, pasta salad, meatless chili (use beans), vegetable sushi...it's a big list! Also, does your mom/dad ever whine about how your family always eats the same fifteen or so dinners, just in rotation? Mine did. If they do, the next time they say that, mention that cooking vegan dinners for the family would definitely be adding variety!

Translation #2: I'm seeing if you're really committed to this. If you heave a sigh and make do with eating what little of your family's meals are cruelty-free, you show your family that vegan eating is hard and not nutritious, that you aren't willing to learn to cook, that veganism means deprival, and a host of other bad things. If you volunteer to cook for yourself and, if need be, buy vegan groceries for yourself (and really do both of those things), you're showing your family that veganism means enough to you for you to take time, effort, and money of your own in order to be happy as a vegan, and you really are dedicated to being vegan. And once they see that you're serious about veganism, your parents will most likely be willing to at least cook for you now and then and chip in for, if not pay for entirely, your vegan groceries.

"I don't get it."

This is often a simple concern some parents have—they might be willing to let you go vegan, they might have accepted that you won't become a frail, sickly, yellowed weakling, they might have bought you this book, but they might not understand just why you want to go vegan and may be merely curious. Explain to them your reasons—no need to go into grisly detail about the ins and outs of factory farms, but it would be worth mentioning that dairy cows and laying hens are still treated cruelly, exploited for their product, still get slaughtered in the end, and so forth. Most parents can understand the reasons for being vegetarian, but many people still live under the impression that dairy and eggs let animals live relatively happy and free lives, which couldn't be further from the truth. You could also mention the environmental or health reasons for a vegan lifestyle.

"Couldn't you just eat free-range?"

This is an attempt by a well-meaning parent to strike a compromise with you—they don't have to cook vegan or worry about where you get such-and-such nutrient, and you get to stamp out animal cruelty in your life, right? Er, *wrong*.

Explain the following (remembering that being respectful, informed, and calm works much better than being angry or judgmental) to your parents: "Free-range" is generally complete mislabeling. The only USDA guideline for an animal food to be called "free-range" is that the animal have mere access to an outside area—it doesn't matter if the animal is given access for an hour of her life and doesn't take it, or if she is crammed outside with hundreds of thousands of her kind and made to stand in her own excrement, etc.—that food will be called free-range even if it was made under virtually the same conditions as a factory farm. It is possible, if sometimes tricky, to find eggs and dairy that were made under humane conditions, yes, but this goes against some of the reasons many people have for being vegan.

Truly free-range animal products still support the idea that animals are here only to serve human needs and desires, completely ignoring the fact that animals are beings with their *own* needs and desires—giving humans their flesh or secretions isn't one of these. Even if they're free-range, animal products are still unhealthy and quite disgusting when you really think about what they are. Cholesterol is cholesterol, breast milk is breast milk, carcinogens are carcinogens, and ovulation is ovulation—it doesn't matter if the animal spent his life in a factory farm or frolicking in a pasture.

Lastly, there's just no way around the fact that using any sort of animal products causes animals to die. Even if a chicken spends her life on the most pleasant and humane farm in the world, there's no special field for her to go once her body stops being able to lay eggs. She goes to slaughter. It doesn't sound nice, but it's true—since it's just throwing away money, it would be economically impossible for a farm to pay for the space, food, and care an animal needs for the years after she's productive and economically wasteful not to sell her for meat after she dies, even if she were to die of natural causes.

The same is true for cows, too—plus dairy means veal. Like all other mammals, a cow gives milk for her baby, right? Just because the milk goes to a human doesn't mean there's no calf. And it doesn't matter whether the calf is male or female—he or she still dies, sex only determines when. Either she'll become a dairy cow and go to slaughter after she's productive, or he'll be veal. Again, it doesn't matter if it's the picture-perfect example of a free-range family farm—economics make these events certain. Thus, even if you don't buy meat, if you buy other animal products, you're still giving the meat industry your support.

"We can't afford for you to be vegan."
So many people assume that vegan diets are inherently more expensive than standard American ones. If you buy nothing but mock meats and soy ice cream, yeah, it's probably going to cost you more. But vegetables, fruits, grains, and beans tend to be cheaper than animal products. So if most of your meals are from fresh produce, legumes, and similar foods, you can probably afford to splurge on some fake meat every now and again. It balances out!

"You live under my roof; you'll follow my rules."
This reaction is typically just another one in disguise. Very, very few parents that have seen that veganism is healthy, that it costs about the same as an omnivorous diet, etc. are going to put a ban on it just because. Try to get your parent to talk with you about what's really up, and then tackle whatever issue is underlying.

Parents often see veganism as complicated, and, yeah, it probably *would* be easier if you ate the same way as the rest of your family, but that doesn't mean that ease trumps everything. Like always, do your homework and show that you know what you're talking about, that you have definite, important reasons for wanting to be vegan beyond to piss off Mom and Dad.

When worst comes to worst, they can't exactly force animal products down your throat. If you've talked with your parents, if you've been calm and informed and mature and everything else, and they still don't like the idea...give it time. If at *all* possible, take charge of your own meals—this shows both that you're serious about going vegan and that it's really not that difficult.

And if they still won't budge? Bring out the big guns. Haven't your parents always raised you to fight for what's right and what you believe in? Don't you want them to be there for you when you need their support? Parents can't argue with that, and when people can't argue, they're forced to actually discuss.

Other things to note:

★ Don't tell your parents anything like, "I'm going to be vegan for my entire life and do *so* much good for the animals and convert so many people to veganism and marry a nice vegan and have vegan children and even when I'm an old person I'll just gum my tofu and be a happy vegan!," even if you fully plan on doing all of that. It'll freak them out.

★ Even if your other family members are eating cheese-covered meat with a side of eggs and a tall glass of milk, eat your vegan meal with them if they want you to. Yes, you'll probably be grossed out by their food, but just try not to concentrate on it. I have so much trouble with this, but if you refuse to eat with them, you make it seem like you're detaching yourself, like you *can't* eat with them, like disrupting the family dinner is something your veganism makes you do. Just because you're eating something different doesn't mean you can't (or shouldn't) eat dinner with your family when they want you to. Plus, if you don't eat with them, they can't ooh and ahh over your food!

∗ The dinner table is never the place to get angry or give a lecture. Seeing your family participate in the cruelty you're very much against can be angering, yes, but save those conversations (not attacks) for later. Talking about such things as people are consuming animals makes them feel judged and puts them on the defensive—neither of which do anything for changing minds. This goes for all people, not just your family.

Just remember that parents are people, too. No matter how frustrating it might get, try to imagine where they're coming from (not only is that a sign of maturity but it gives you a better idea of how to present your case!). If you want them to really discuss something with you and not just force you to live with their opinion on something, you've got to do the same. Show that you're looking for a mature conversation rather than an argument and that, even though you stand your ground, you are willing to talk.

Chapter Two: Friends and Peers

Teenagers are a tricky bunch. Because we're so young, our impressions of how things are "supposed" to be are not as deep set, so we're the group most open to alternative lifestyles and to changing our own lifestyles. But, also because we're so young, we sometimes have difficulty seeing beyond what's directly in front of us (on our plates), the larger effects our actions have, and we're more tied to the way food tastes. This can be reeeeally frustrating when you're a teenager, yet you've seen beyond and gone vegan and all, and you're wondering why other people your age can't grow up and do the same.

Usually when teenagers come to you about your veganism, they are simply curious. Either they don't know what vegan means, or they want to know what you really eat, or why you went vegan, etc. Curiosity is a good thing. It means they practically come up to you and beg for vegan outreach! No, really. If somebody doesn't know a thing about veganism (remembering that you have to know something about what you're teasing someone about), they're probably going to cover all the bases with their questions and give you plenty of opportunity to be the best advocate for veganism you can be. Sometimes, that is.

Other times, they're counting on you to be an easy target to make fun of. People look for differences to point out, heighten, and put in a negative light, and veganism is definitely a difference. They know you're going to be in a bothered and awkward position when they tell you, in great detail, about whatever dairy orgy they've just had.

They also might not assume that you have actual reason for being vegan, don't know much about it, and are going to be tripped up by their oh-so-original (har) stupid questions.

Like parents (well, and everybody), teenagers, whether they're curious and nice or mean and uninterested, are best dealt with in a calm, educated, nonconfrontational manner.

If they're curious...

Educate 'em! At least initially, though, be somewhat vague about it. Saying something like "For ethical reasons" or "Well, dairy cows and laying hens are treated the same way and still become meat in the end" and easing into the specifics as they ask more is going to get you a better response than being vegangelical about it and preaching about battery cages and bolt guns. Going for the first option allows the non-vegan to set the pace for how much you tell them and how fast. Then they're just interested, not overwhelmed. The wheels start turnin' then—if you go for the second option, those wheels turn off completely.

If somebody asks you a simple question about why you didn't just settle on being vegetarian and you whip out your soapbox and start screeching about why they're a horrible, vile person for supporting animal exploitation, that person is going to feel judged and overwhelmed. Once they're on the defensive, forget about it—nobody's going to be receptive to what you're trying to say if you're doing it by attacking their way of life. You weren't always vegan, correct? If someone had marched up to you, shoved a picture of a bloody pig in your face, and began screaming about the horrors of factory farms, would you have gone vegan sooner? No. Inundated with new and unhappy information, you'd simply be overwhelmed and probably be even further set in your ways. Plus, people like that make all vegans seem psychotic, and the vast majority of us are completely normal people who simply decided to live an ethical lifestyle and be vegan.

If they're confused...

Set them straight, nicely. Someone who wants to know what vegans eat but doesn't is one thing. Someone who is certain that vegans eat fish and cheese and gelatin is quite another. The more of those people there are, the more likely it is that you or another vegan is going to be fed something not vegan accidentally, or that someone's going to "go vegan" and still eat fish, et cetera. None of those people are good. They're only going to make things frustrating for you sometime, so you might as well make sure they know what's what. Remember, though, nonconfrontationally ease into it and end with something positive that doesn't make them feel like an idiot. For example, if someone mentions that Jell-O is vegan, you could say "Well, Jell-O is made with gelatin, which isn't vegan, but they do make vegan jello with different ingredients."

If your friends think you're going to change drastically...

When you go make the big life change that going vegan is, it's not uncommon for your friends to assume that you're going to turn into a punk, hippie, Mr./Ms. PETA, or some other vegan stereotype (not that there's anything wrong with punks or hippies). They might expect you to start marching up to trees and breathing in their life aura, or to start all your sentences with, "Well, PETA said..." and they might be worried about "losing you." Like a parent who thinks veganism is just a phase, this one can really only be solved with time. Show your friends that you're the same person you've always been...just vegan. In time they'll see that you're your same old awesome self. If they really believe you're going to become a different person and you're really tired of it, make a special effort to act like you usually do. Hang out with your friends in the same places, listen to the same music with them, tell the same kinds of jokes, etc. Even if you've been listening to a lot of Rise Against lately, or have been noticing that you feel really connected to the world since going veg, or are really digging PETA's fact sheets, don't mention it to your friends, at least not for a while, if you're that worried.

If they think plants feel pain...

Oh, no. Not the plants. Bring up veganism and omnivores immediately reveal their true colors as champions of the oppressed and downtrodden: plants! They'll be intent on showing you how you have to either eat meat and dairy and eggs or eat nothing at all to be ethically consistent. Yeesh, people are fun. Here's the thing: plants have neither central nervous systems nor pain receptors. When you try and cause a human or nonhuman animal pain, they scream, make a face, or react in some way. When you try and cause a plant pain...nothing happens. Even if, by some stretch of the imagination, plants felt pain or suffered when they died, veganism would still be the better choice. To eat plant products, you eat the plant directly. To eat animal products, first you feed plants (often several pounds of them, per pound of animal product) to the animal and then eat the animal. So, if you're vegan, you're still murdering fewer poor, defenseless, innocent plants than you would if you were a vegetarian or an omnivore.

If they think you can't "take a joke"...
Have an omni ask you a completely unoriginal, asinine question, give them an answer (isn't that the point of asking a question?), and all of a sudden, you have absolutely no sense of humor. Or that's what the omni would have you think, at least. If you're feeling particularly ballsy, make a joke back and then ask them why *they* can't take a joke. However, I don't really advise this, as it can backfire. Just ask them (nicely) why they asked a question if they didn't want an answer, or, if they were kidding, why they didn't say they were.

If they make fun of you...
Do what you've always been told: ignore it because they're only trying to get a rise out of you and if you don't react they'll stop and blah, blah, blah. It's true. If you freak out every time someone suggests that you live off iceberg lettuce and veggie burgers, it's going to be funny to them. They'll keeping doing it and it will only get worse, so you're best off just ignoring it the first time.

Use witty remarks and comebacks at your own risk. If you've thought of a good one and really want to use it, go ahead, but know that they can backfire horribly and make you (and therefore your decision to be vegan) look stupid. If you absolutely have to, try to think like an omni who's desperate to make you look bad beforehand. If you really can't think of any way they could possibly twist your retort against you, fire away.

You getting made fun of for being vegan really depends two things. One of these is simply the school you go to. For example, in all the time I've been vegan, no one's ever teased me. I've gotten stupid questions, sure, but no one's ever made it their mission to make me feel bad about being veg or said things to deliberately get a rise out of me (siblings excluded). On the other hand, I've heard of vegan teenagers getting chicken bones left on their desks and other idiotic things. In the latter case, try acting like you're unaffected by it at first and see if it stops. If they keep doing it, yes, confront them about it. Be reasonably civil, at least at first. Just because they're immature doesn't mean you have to be. The second thing that impacts whether or not you get made fun of is how you let the world know you're vegan. The normal-seeming vegan who is hesitant to vegangelize but not to share their great food and explain about things when appropriate is going to get a vastly different response than the self-alienating vegan who is quick to give others lectures about factory farming and what murderers other people are, between bites of iceberg lettuce. For the most part, vegans that seem nice are treated nicely, or, at least, nicer than the scary vegans are treated.

If they give excuses for not being vegan...

Gah, this is annoying. On one hand, if you resist the urge to scream, and just smile and nod along, you make it seem like their lame excuses are valid reasons for not being vegan. On the other, if you tell them why they're wrong straight up, you're going to seem preachy.

I think the best way to deal with this is to remind them that you were once just the same as they were, but you changed, and that people don't come into the world with a birthmark in the shape of a "V" on their butt or anything. For instance, if they make a comment along the lines of "I would be vegan, but I have no self-control," it would be good to say something like "Yeah, I thought it was going to take a lot of willpower, but it really didn't... I lost the taste for animal products pretty quickly, especially after I found out about [such-and-such animal cruelty]." Or, if they say they would be vegan but they would miss such-and-such, say that you thought you would miss it a lot, but you just had the vegan version and you didn't miss it at all. No matter what you say, just establish that you were once in the same spot they are but now you're (obviously) vegan, and make sure you make known whatever caused you to think differently, whether it was a book, a vegan ice cream, a simple realization, whatever.

If they apologize for eating meat/dairy/eggs...

Non-vegans often think that because you're vegan, you're going to take offense at people around you eating animal products. While having people nearby consuming such foods may bother you somewhat, non-vegans will frequently think that they're committing some crime against you and need to apologize for it. And when they do apologize, it is awkward. You don't want to say, "Oh, it's fine," but you also don't want to go into some diatribe about factory farms. So what do you do? I usually just tell people that my choices are mine and their choices are theirs. It implies that you have definite reason for being vegan but doesn't make others feel attacked or judged. Simple as that. If you're feeling gutsy or really want to get people thinking, say it's not your funeral or ask them to not apologize to you.

Pick your battles. Sometimes people are being genuine, and then it's worth it to talk to them. Other times, people are just trying to get a rise out of you, and any attempts at changing their mind will only frustrate you. Do what you feel comfortable with—when I first went vegan I thought it was my duty to tell all I knew about veganism to anyone who raised an eyebrow, and I felt like a bad vegan if I didn't. Now, I know I don't have to bother with people who are just being stupid. People often make stupid comments to try to justify their consumption of animals to themselves, and chiming in is rarely worth your time.

Chapter Three: Yourself

You're just inches away from being vegan. Inches. You know that dairy cows and laying hens are treated just as horribly as other animals and still become meat in the end. You know that it isn't cool to treat sentient beings like objects. You know that you can go vegan and still be healthy and eat yummy things. You know all the other reasons why veganism rocks. But what if there's just a leeettle something holding you back? Whatever it is, no matter how small or stupid, it's stopping you from being vegan, and that makes it big and important and in need of being dealt with. Behold Chapter 3, which is also useful for using a reverse-psychology kind of thing on people who are 50 percent human and 50 percent excuse.

I don't know how to cook!

Let's break this one down. You don't know how to make food. What are you eating now, then? If this is more of a "my parents won't cook for me" thing, turn to page 37 to deal with that. You might think that your parents will refuse to cook for you and you'll be forced to make every single meal for yourself, but nine times out of ten, that's not the case. Your parents might not be willing to cook vegan meals for you every single night, though, so you really should learn how to cook. Plus, cooking really is a lot of fun! There's such a difference between a meal that's right in front of you and a meal that you made, a bunch of ingredients that you combined in just such a way to make a delicious meal. Eating it feels different and good, and you feel productive and like you can take care of yourself.

If you aren't used to cooking whatsoever, start off with some things that aren't recipes but still require minimal preparation. Think boxed things—mac 'n' cheeze (like Road's End), couscous (like Near East), Asian (like Simply Asia). Those don't really count as cooking but they'll get you used to following steps, as in a recipe, and performing the simplest of cooking tasks.

After you've mastered all that, ease into some easy recipes and get a hang of those. Simple pasta dishes, one-pot dishes, and things like that are great places to start. Try and experiment with one new cooking method or one new food every week—this is a great, great way to expand both your culinary skills and the variety of your diet. Never tried Mediterranean food? Spend a week incorporating foods like hummus, falafel, and pita bread into your meals. Don't know how to sauté? Plan dinners with the addition of sautéed veggies or tofu.

It's not that hard. Prevegan, I didn't really know much about cooking. I could make cookies and boil water for pasta, but that was about it. I didn't really like stepping outside of the things that I knew how to make already. Going vegan varied my diet a lot, but it increased my ability as a cook a lot, too. Now, I love to experiment in the kitchen with different foods and spices. Once I tried marinating some tempeh without a recipe, and it was gross—way too salty! But one of my favorite recipes, Veghettios (page 125) was created simply by throwing things into a pot on a whim. It's definitely a process of trial and error, but when a recipe does work out, it's worth it.

A great list of vegan cookbooks can be found in Chapter 5.

I could never give up cheese!
Cheese is tough for a lot of people to give up. Even when you've phased all other animal products out of your diet, cheese can be the one thing holding you back. But there's actual reason for this—cheese is a drug! Mmhmm. Cheese's main protein, casein (found irritatingly often in some nondairy cheeses), breaks

down during digestion to form compounds similar to morphine called casomorphins. The reason for this, class, is that milk is supposed to be given to calves from their moms. The casomorphins are intended to draw that calf back to the mother's udders so the calf will keep drinking the milk and grow up. Instead, casomorphins give your stomach and brain a relaxed, slightly drowsy feeling (it's called "comfort food" for a reason) and draw you back to the fridge.

So what can you do to break the addiction? What I think is most effective is thinking of how that cheese got to you. Don't think that you're a horrible person for eating cheese, just think about how that cheese came to your plate. Think about a cow on her way to be artificially impregnated against her will. Think about that same cow moaning and wailing months later when her child is taken away from her. Think about that calf chained in a crate in the dark, and ask yourself, is it really worth it? If thinking about this makes you feel like you're guilt-tripping yourself, why? Are the ten or twenty minutes of pleasure you'll get from the cheese worth the hours and hours and hours of suffering put into it? (By the way, this approach works for whatever other food, if any, is keeping you back.) I mean, think of it this way. It would be nice to have someone to do all your work for you so you could just relax all day. But are you going to force a black person to do this because they are black? Of course not. Your ethical problems with slavery outweigh your desire to have someone do everything for you. Cheese is the same way. Yeah, it might taste good, but your ethical problems with the slavery and commodification of sentient beings trump your desire to just have a "normal" pizza. Plus, cheese is nothing more than the breast milk of some animal fermented with certain bacteria to make it solidify. Yummy.

Vegan cheeses can be a tad frustrating, since a lot of nondairy cheeses with "soy" and "cheeze" in the name contain casein, which is still an animal product and therefore not vegan. Look for brands that specifically say vegan on the package, such as Daiya (my favorite),

Cheezly, or Follow Your Heart. The world of vegan cheese is a fast-paced one. When I first started writing this book in 2007, vegan cheese was either readily available but kind of odd-tasting, or delicious and hard to find (like, only-in-Europe hard). Now, though, that isn't the case. Daiya, for example, really tastes like dairy cheese (even my omnivorous family likes it), melts and gets stringy like dairy cheese, and is sold in every Whole Foods store (and other places as well) throughout the nation. There are all different kinds of vegan cheese from shreds to slices to spreads in every flavor from bacon (really) to Monterey Jack, and trying different brands to find out which you like best is no longer a treacherous, plastic-tasting labyrinth. It only takes about three weeks for you to grow new tastebuds (and thus for new tastes to become normal to you), too.

It would be too weird!

Yeah, caring about animals and wanting to live by your ethics is way too weird. No, I know what you mean—veganism is probably the most socially difficult when you're a teenager than at any other time, but then again that's probably true of just about everything. If you really, truly want to be vegan, know you can, know you should—then is being yourself really that weird? Weird enough for you to hide it and pretend to be something else? Sometimes, yeah, being vegan is weird. It's not always fun asking the waitstaff at restaurants the exact ingredients in a food. It's not always fun being asked if you would drink milk if it magically started raining from the sky. But when it comes down to it, it's worth it. Don't sell out.

And you know what? You're going to be pleasantly surprised, sometimes. When I first went vegan, I was scared that the only conversations with my friends and classmates about my veganism would be to the tune of "Animals don't feel pain but broccoli does and that's why you fail at life." However, most of the conversations I've had about veganism have been pretty positive. A lot of times, people are purely curious and pretty decent, and the interested people who think it's cool definitely outweigh the oh-so-original losers who try and make their way of life look superior to yours. It's also not uncommon for me to tell people I'm vegan and hear, "Yeah, my brother's a vegan," or, "Oh, have you ever eaten at this place? They have great tofu." When I first went vegan my brothers liked to badger me about it, and while they still occasionally do this, one of my brothers recently made vegan cupcakes for me, and they were delicious. There are a lot of good people out there, so have some faith in them.

Wouldn't being a strict vegetarian be the same thing?

For about a month before I actually went vegan, I was a strict vegetarian—I would never down a glass of milk or dig into an omelet but I was totally fine with eating something processed that contained whey or a muffin made with egg. This was partially because of my parents—I was worried that if they knew I was avoiding *all* animal products intentionally, they would force me to eat them, so I thought I would be consuming fewer animal products total if I ate the small things willingly, but partially because I just didn't see how the tiny things added up to any amount of significance. Well, they do—it might not really matter if only *you* eat a drop of whey, but imagine if a thousand people thought it didn't matter, and ate it. Then it would definitely matter. If you don't think it really would, why would did you want to go vegan? You on your own are not going to bring down the entire animal agriculture industry. It's your belief that you are part of a chain reaction and a group of people who, though they don't know each other, are making a difference that makes you do anything, right? If somebody went vegan before you, and then you, and somebody after you, and somebody after that, and so on, that's what's going to make a difference. You believe that or you wouldn't be vegan. So couldn't that concept go the other way? If you think some marginal animal ingredient isn't that big of a deal, and keep eating it, and someone does after you, and someone after them... it will add up, and not in the good way like veganism.

I like to go out to eat!

Hey, that makes two of us! While there will be restaurants that will frustrate you, you can get a plate of food just about anywhere if you're just willing to ask the server a few questions. Most restaurants are pretty accommodating, especially if you say you "can't have" a food rather than that you "don't eat" it. Saying that you can't have something implies that, if they feed it to you, your face will swell up and you will break out in hives and then die and then sue them. In that order. Lots of restaurants have websites that allow you to scope out how vegan-friendly their menu is in advance, and if you have an mp3 player, it's easy to find guides to vegan options at chain restaurants and put them in as text files.

You may be surprised how veg-friendly your city is. For example, my hometown is Kansas City, the heart of the Midwest and one of the barbeque capitals of the nation. Doesn't sound very veg-friendly, does it? Before I searched online for "Kansas City vegan" and became involved with my local veg*n (that's vegan/vegetarian) group, I just assumed that there wasn't that much in town for me to eat. How wrong I was! KC has a pizza parlor that offers vegan mozzarella, an Indian restaurant with an extensive vegan menu, some great vegan brunch, multiple Chinese restaurants with large vegan sections of the menu, and even an entirely vegan restaurant complete with raw food and cashew-based ice cream, plus tons of other veg-friendly restaurants. You may assume that because you don't live in a travel destination, there's nothing for you, but you may be wrong. Poke around both online and in the real world—if a menu doesn't have much, you can always leave. You'll never know what great vegan meals are waiting to be eaten until you go looking for them.

Even if you don't have restaurants with specific vegan menus, there are certain kinds of restaurants that tend to have more vegan options than others, namely ethnic ones. Thai, Chinese, Mediterranean, Japanese, Indian, and Mexican restaurants are usually more vegan-friendly than plain ol' American ones, though there are still some things you need to watch for. At Thai restaurants, beware of hidden fish sauces and fish oils (just ask your server to leave them out) and note that menus sometimes do not say that there is egg in Pad Thai, so ask. Chinese restaurants, unless they specify that it is vegetarian/vegan, sometimes use ground pork in their Ma Po Tofu.

Mediterranean restaurants are pretty straightforward unless you're worried about, say, your falafel being cooked on the same grill as a piece of meat, and even then you can simply voice your concerns to your server. When you think Japanese restaurants, you probably think sushi, but there is definitely veggie sushi out there waiting to be eaten. Indian restaurants sometimes cook their dishes with ghee (a liquid product from butter), but you can ask your server if the restaurant does this, and they'd be happy to cook your dish with vegetable oil instead. Mexican restaurants sometimes use lard in their beans or cook rice in chicken broth, but again, just ask.

I can't care about animal rights enough to go vegan—human rights/anticapitalism/feminism/other issues come first!

Whether you're a champion for a woman's right to choose or against world hunger, you automatically rock. But if you want to rock even more, think about being vegan. As I see it, every kind of injustice is related at some level. Veganism was my first foray into social justice, but once I started caring about animal rights it was hard not to start caring about human rights, too. The more I found out about factory farming, the more I realized that it's not just something that affects the lives of cows and chickens. Meatpacking is a low-skill, high-risk job—Human Rights Watch has called it the most dangerous factory job in America. The human workers in factory farms are frequently undocumented immigrants who work with no health care or job security. Even if they are legal citizens, that doesn't make the job any safer. The U.S. Department of Labor's Bureau of Labor Statistics shows that almost one in three slaughterhouse workers suffers from illness or injury every year, in comparison to one in ten workers in other manufacturing jobs. Killing lines move incredibly fast (more animals per hour, more money per hour) and this is often a source of injury to workers. Buying safety gear or slowing the line costs profit. Like with animals, it's cheaper to replace an employee than it is to give an injured one proper health care. Injured workers can rarely afford full health care on their salaries—which also cease once they take time from work to heal. For more information on this subject, read *Slaughterhouse* by Gail Eisnitz or *Fast Food Nation* by Eric Schlosser.

Likewise, the oppression of women and animals are very much tied together—the same principle that allows a sexist to see a woman as an object at worst or second-class citizen at best, rather than an intelligent and capable sister, daughter, and friend is what allows a speciesist to see only a hamburger or an emotionless milk-giving automaton rather than a living, feeling being. For more, read Carol Adams's amazing book *The Sexual Politics of Meat*. I could go on and on, but the point is that there is no kind of oppression that stands alone in the world. I'm not saying that you have to care about every issue equally and work for them to the same degree, but is this a genuine ethical dilemma? How are you helping humans by continuing to eat animals? Is eating chickpeas instead of chicken such an incredible effort that you lose all your time and ability to fight for human rights? You don't have to liberate every single oppressed being in the world overnight, but you also shouldn't wear blinders.

Part Two:
Stuff You Should Know

If you've just gone vegan (congratulations!), there's probably a lot you're wondering. You might know why eating dairy is ethically wrong, but how do you make up for the calcium you used to get from dairy? Having just gone vegan, you're all afire with excitement and want to spread your excitement to the world but don't know how to go about it. You might not want to eat the flesh of a chicken, but you've lived your whole life enjoying the taste...what to do? You're vegan now, but your biology class is dissecting frogs next month. Who are some important vegans you should know about? It seems as if all of your makeup and toiletries are tested on animals—help! Behold, dear reader, part deux!

CHAPTER FOUR: HEALTH AND NUTRITION

★

Tell someone you're vegan, or even thinking about becoming vegan, and one of the first questions you'll get will be about health. After all, eating a vegan diet means cutting out three categories of food that most people see as major. It's no wonder other people think that all vegans are a sickly shade of pale yellow with dull hair and broken nails, barely energized enough to shake our protest signs with our pencil-thin wrists. From your mom being worried you'll stop eating anything and wither away, to a well-meaning aunt gifting you with a massive jar of multivitamins lest you fall over and die, from a teacher giving you an article about the dangers of being anywhere near soy, to being asked "Where do you get your protein?" by every single person you meet, you had better be prepared to let the world know that the vegan diet is just as healthy as whatever crazy meal plan everyone else is on, if not healthier. And not only do you have to know what to tell people when they ask about the state of your body, you have to actually be healthy!

Fear not, because a well-planned plant-based diet is pretty much the healthiest one there is.* Once you know where to get all your nutrients and everything, blowing

---

* FYI, cutting out animal products does not mean you're automatically going to be Mr./Ms. Health. Eat your veggies!

the jaundiced-vegan-weakling idea out of the water is easy as pie (mmm, pie). A vegan diet is filled with the same calcium, protein, and iron as omni/vegetarian diets, with more fiber, zero cholesterol (cholesterol is produced in the liver, and plants obviously don't have livers), less saturated fat, more antioxidants...basically, more of the good stuff, less of the bad stuff.

So why is the vegan diet so healthy? After all, diets containing meat, dairy, and eggs have been pushed upon us since infancy as the paradigm of balance and health. Wouldn't the most widespread diet be the healthiest? Yes, but, looking at all humans in all parts of the world in all periods of time, a plant-based diet *is* the most common. Diets heavy in animal products, like the Western diet you're most used to, have only arisen in the past few centuries—this is due mainly to the Industrial Revolution and the rise of factory farming. As factory farming came about, more meat, dairy, and eggs could be produced than with more traditional and less intensive methods. The more animal products that were available, the more were bought. When harvests failed, animal products were the most calorie-dense thing to eat available, and what kept people from starving. But, for the most part, our society now is definitely not starving (America is the most obese nation in the world!) and animal products are certainly not necessary for staying alive (or for enjoying your food or eating what's convenient, for that matter).

The fact that diets featuring animal products have been supported and recommended by the USDA is largely political rather than scientific. The USDA started off in the late 1800s with the purpose of assisting farmers with their surplus produce. As many of those farmers moved to animal-based agriculture, they maintained a heavy influence on the USDA and its actions throughout the next century, especially regarding the creation of the four basic food groups in 1956 and the food pyramid in 1992. Today, lobbyists from the meat and dairy industries still play a major role in the USDA.

But I digress. Ish. Anyway, just because you can survive on one diet doesn't mean you can thrive on it. Personally, my health didn't change at all in going from omnivore to vegetarian, but I've noticed a really positive change in my health since going vegan. My skin is much clearer, I have more energy during the day, I fall asleep faster at night, and I used to have some digestive issues that resolved themselves entirely once I dropped the animal products. I don't remember the last time I had the flu, and my colds are much shorter. I had hit a plateau in my growth, but I've grown another inch since going vegan. Before I was vegan, I was anemic and underweight and now I'm neither of those things. Overall, I just feel healthier.

The reason diets featuring animal products are so unhealthy is basically the animal proteins they contain. Animal protein, at any level of consumption, greatly contributes to atherosclerosis (fatty buildup in arteries), kidney disease, high cholesterol (which in turn can lead to heart attacks), and calcium extraction from the bones (*The Vegan Sourcebook*). Animal protein is more effective at raising cholesterol than both saturated fat intake and dietary cholesterol (Campbell and Campbell, *The China Study* [Dallas: BenBella Books, 2005]). High cholesterol and other heart problems are being thought of as normal health problems that simply come with age—they aren't! They're only normal for people who eat animal protein. I mean, think about it. Vegan diets are completely free of cholesterol and animal protein. A lifetime of eating lots more cholesterol than you need (your liver makes all that's necessary) and any amount of animal protein (especially in the amounts most Westerners eat it) is going to add up. Fun fact, heart disease and other "normal problems" start in childhood—they just might not rear their ugly heads until adulthood.

Also, dairy is a joke. Dairy products do nothing to stave off osteoporosis, and actually increase the risk of bone fracture. This, again, has to do with the animal protein in milk, cheese, yogurt, and other dairy products. For example, The Harvard Nurses' Health Study, which followed more than seventy-five thousand women for twelve years, showed no protective effect of greater consumption of dairy on fracture risk—increased intake of calcium from dairy products was actually associated with a higher fracture risk. Fractures are often used to measure osteoporosis. Another example of the animal protein-calcium relationship was shown in John Robbins's book *Diet for a New America*. The Bantu women of Africa consume a mere 350 mg of calcium per day and very little protein, and are able to breastfeed their many children, never become calcium-deficient and rarely break a bone or lose a tooth, while the Inuit, who consume around 2,000 mg of calcium and at least 250 g of protein a day, have one of the world's highest rates of osteoporosis.

Dairy products also raise the risk of many kinds of cardiovascular disease, diabetes, and cancer, especially ovarian and prostate. A milk sugar is broken down by the body into another sugar, and this sugar can build up in the blood, causing ovarian and other cancers. Women who consume dairy on a regular basis can have up to three times the risk of ovarian cancer as other women. Hey teenage girls, does this sound like a habit you want to be getting into? Dairy products also contain high levels of antibiotics, hormones, and pesticides (The Physicians' Committee for Responsible Medicine, "What's Wrong With Dairy?").

For much more information on the health detriments of an omnivorous or vegetarian diet, see Books on Health, page 78. Great online resources on vegan health include the website of the Physicians' Committee for Responsible Medicine (www.pcrm.org) and Vegan Outreach's website Vegan Health (www.veganhealth. org). The majority of the information in the following section is derived from Vegan Health, the PCRM, *The China Study* by T. Colin Campbell and Thomas M. Campbell (BenBella Books, 2005), and *The Vegan Sourcebook* by Joanne Stepaniak. These are my favorite, and the best-documented, resources on vegan health.

So now that you know why non-vegan diets are unhealthy, let's talk about how to be (and stay) a healthy vegan. You could probably figure this out, but simply cutting the animal products out of your diet does not make you, by default, the epitome of health. You can't absorb nutrients by thinking about healthy foods and you can't stay healthy by eating a diet of white bread and soda. Read on! Be healthy!

CALCIUM

Far too many people believe that, without products from cow's milk, it's nearly impossible to get calcium. The belief that cow's milk is the only, or at least the best, source of calcium is very ingrained into our society. Nonstop, from teachers, magazine ads, and cows with milk mustaches, the idea that cow's milk = calcium and calcium = cow's milk is forced upon us. So, when somebody goes vegan or even hears of somebody going vegan, ingesting enough calcium seems like a big issue. It's not that they think it's impossible, they just truly do not know sources of calcium that weren't inside a cow at some point.

Truth is, calcium from a cow is *not* the best source of calcium out there—it messes with the acidity of your blood. Animal protein (which is obviously present in a glass of milk) tends to make the blood more acidic, so, to compensate, the body pulls calcium out of the bones and into the blood, neutralizing the acid and encouraging its passage into the urine, along with the calcium. Dairy products do put calcium into your body, sure, but they pull it right back out again.

Calcium from plant sources is absorbed almost twice as well as the calcium in cow's milk, as well as tending to have more calcium per calorie than dairy products. Vegan calcium sources include:
* vegan milks (such as soy, rice, almond, oat, hazelnut, hemp, etc.)
* leafy greens (such as broccoli, kale, chard, collards, etc.—but stick to dark green ones)

* beans (especially white, navy, and great northern)
* calcium-fortified orange juice
* tofu (but make sure it's calcium-set)
* other vegetables like squash and sweet potatoes
* other calcium-fortified foods like granola/ energy bars, cereals, etc.
* other vegan dairy alternatives like soy pudding and rice yogurt

IRON

The American Dietetic Association's Position Paper on Vegetarian Diets has shown that iron deficiency is no more common in vegans than in omnivores. Plus, vitamin C—consumed by vegans at three to four times the amount consumed by omnivores—increases iron absorption. Still, getting enough iron is important for your blood cells—and especially important for teenage girls. Teenagers need between 11.3 and 14.8 mg of iron per day. Vegan iron sources include:

* Legumes like chickpeas, lentils, pistachios, black-eyed peas and cashews
* Sesame seeds/tahini (a paste made from sesame seeds)
* Blackstrap molasses (throw it in a smoothie or baked goods)
* Dried apricots
* Spinach
* Broccoli
* Raisins
* Watermelon
* Many fortified foods, like oatmeal, cereal, and granola/energy bars

PROTEIN

Ah, the protein question. I love this one. Protein is extremely difficult to obtain in vegan diets as it is found exclusively in meat, dairy, and eggs, and absolutely nowhere else. Nowhere. Find a nice protein shake powder you like and make sure to take a lot of it, for without enormous amounts of protein you will shrivel into oblivion and die.

I'm kidding, of course...though that's what most omnivores would have you believe. Does it make any amount of logical sense that protein would be in huge amounts in certain foods and completely absent in all other foods? No, it does not. Protein is in just about every single food, with the exception of oils and a few fruits. If you're getting enough calories, the smaller amounts of protein in those foods will add up to be a totally adequate amount. It also doesn't make sense that you need incredibly large amounts of protein to stay healthy—to figure out how much you need, multiply your body weight by .36, and that's how many grams you need in a day. One gram of protein has four calories, so you really don't need as much as you think. Let's say you weigh 125 lb., need 45 g of protein a day, and eat 2,500 calories a day. Only 180 of those calories—a mere 7 percent—need to be from protein. See? You don't need enormous slabs of steak to stay healthy.

For a long time it was thought that, in vegetarian diets, protein had to be carefully combined in order to get the proper balance of amino acids. Not true. Different foods contain different amino acids, yes, but your body stores these and draws upon them as needed. The American Dietetic Association states in their *Position Paper on Vegetarian Diets*: "Plant sources of protein alone can provide adequate amounts of essential amino acids if a variety of plant foods are consumed and energy needs are met. Research suggests that complementary proteins do not need to be consumed at the same time and that consumption of various sources of amino acids over the course of the day should ensure adequate nitrogen retention and use in healthy persons." As long as you're one of the rare vegans eating things other than lentils and sticks (har, har!), and as long as you're consuming all the calories you need, you'll be set on protein. I make a daily effort to get all the calcium, B12, and so forth that I need, but I honestly do not think about protein one bit. It's like worrying about getting enough air—if you aren't, something is very, very wrong with the way you live your life, so don't worry about it. For example, a typical day of eating for me might look like this: I have some cereal and fruit with a glass of soymilk for breakfast, rice and veggies and vegan chicken strips with peanut sauce for lunch, a burrito and a glass of orange juice for dinner, and an apple and another glass of soymilk for an evening snack. Without thinking about it at all, I have consumed enough calories and enough protein to keep me goin' for another day.

Pretty much every vegan food you think up contains protein, but these are especially high in it:
* beans and other legumes, like lentils
* nuts and nut butters
* tofu, tempeh, and seitan
* soymilk, soy yogurt, and other soy products

B12

If you only read one part of this section, read this! B12 is the one nutrient that you really, really must make sure you have a constant and definite source of. Deficiency in B12 can cause irreversible damage to your nervous system, and the nervous system is a wondrous thing. Years and years and years ago, before we had filled up the earth's soil with lots of chemicals and pesticides, B12 was found naturally in soil. So, when people ate plants, they could get B12 both from the plants themselves and from the soil still left on the plants. However, today even organic fruits, vegetables, and grains are grown in soil without B12, making animal products the most common source for B12. But, if you're vegan, don't worry! You can still get your B12 from a variety of sources. There is no unfortified plant source of B12, but because it is made by bacterial fermentation (and bacteria are obviously not in the animal kingdom), there are fortified vegan sources of B12. These include supplements, soymilk, nutritional yeast, cereals, and more. Just make sure that you have a consistent source of it. Different brands of different foods contain different amounts of B12. For example, most brands of soymilk will give you all the B12 you need in two glasses, but some random brands aren't fortified with it because they are made by fools. As such, it's best to rely on more than one source to make absolutely certain that you're getting enough (and it's not like omnis are getting their B12 from only one source, either). If you're taking a supplement that's strictly B12, get 10–100 mcg (that's .01–.1 percent of a milligram) a day.

OMEGAS

Omega-3 and omega-6 fatty acids are polyunsaturated fatty acids that aid in heart and brain health as well as benefiting your immune and developmental systems. While you do have to focus on having them in your diet at all, you also want to make sure you're getting them in proportion to each other. Ideally, you should consume three to five times the amount of omega-6 as you do of omega-3. One of the most annoying things you'll hear from fish-eating "vegetarians" (really, pescetarians) is that they just *have* to eat fish so that they'll get their omega-3 and omega-6 fatty acids. Guess what, pesky pesces? The fish don't even make the omegas themselves. They get it from the algae—a plant!—that they eat. Be like the fishies and eat plants...though, lucky for you, there are much tastier sources of omegas than algae. These include:

* fortified foods like soymilk
* kiwis
* ground flaxseeds (and they must be ground for proper absorption) and flaxseed oil—shoot for a tablespoon of seeds or a teaspoon of oil
* walnuts
* There are also vegan omega-3/-6 supplements available.

Other nutrition-related stuff:

CALORIES

Getting enough calories on a vegan diet really isn't an issue, but I think I should address it so the worried parents of aspiring vegan youth will stop their worrying. It is true that plant products tend to be lower in calories than animal products, but a vegan diet does not mean you stop eating and turn into a skeleton. If you really think your child is going vegan as a way to restrict what they eat, sit down and talk to them about why they wants to be vegan and let them go vegan for a few weeks. If they only eat dry salad and multivitamins, there might be a problem. If the amount of food they eats stays the same, if they're getting enough veggies and fruits and whole grains but still eating normally and including healthy fat—like in peanut butter or olive oil, for instance—in their diet, hooray! You've got a smart child on your hands. Personally? I'm a teenage girl of average weight and I gained a few pounds going vegan, but I'm still at a healthy weight. When I first made the switch, I wasn't sure if the desserts would be all that great, so I thought I would try making some...ohhh, were they great. Hence, a few pounds. I also eat more, eat a wider variety of food, and usually eat healthier since going vegan. I still love a cupcake or two or some chips, but I also like the taste of vegetables better now and am more conscious of what I'm putting into my body, so it balances out. Hey, vegan hopefuls, you know what's great about being vegan? When you do gain weight you're not gaining weight, you're just doing your part to defy the stereotype of the skin-and-bones vegan!

VARIETY

Eating a varied diet is important for so many reasons. When you eat the same stuff over and over and over again, it gets boring. Even if there are a few foods in particular that you love and just have to have all the time, change things up and make it more exciting! Do you just looove couscous? Make it with these spices this time and serve it with vegan chicken strips. Change the spices the next time and plop some roasted vegetables on it. Try yet another spice combination and put spinach and cashews on top. Now that you've made such a switch in your diet, it's a great time to add foods into your diet that you've never heard of or have been afraid of trying. Go to page 117 for a list of some awesome foods you may never have tasted before in your life, but can become favorites of yours! Eating a varied diet is also important in showing that vegans live healthy, happy lives. If someone met you and found out that you ate the same seven dinners week after week, would your diet seem that exciting? Nope. But what if you told them about your diet and they were impressed with all the different yummy things you ate? You'd have shown them that vegans are just as happy as the next person, if not more so, and that's a great feeling. Plus, if you only eat certain foods in repetition, you're only getting the nutrients in those foods, so if you're lacking in something, it adds up fast. Don't just drink soymilk—drink ricemilk and almond milk and the other milks out there. Don't just eat lettuce—eat spinach and arugula and kale and chard. Don't just base your meals on the vegan version of something non-vegan...forget the concept of a meal being meat-and-potatoes and try something new that tastes good for what it is, not because of what it's imitating.

BEING A JUNK FOOD VEGAN

You might be vegan now, but you're still a teenager, and that probably means that you would probably rather have potatoes, fried and in the French style, on the side of your meal, not a raw salad. I'm the same way, and so are most people. Fried things are yummy, sugar is yummy, salt is yummy. But, seriously, just try some vegetables that aren't white or slathered in Earth Balance (vegan butter). And while we're talking about white things, remember the importance of getting whole grains—white bread, white rice, and white noodles are really low in fiber and other nutrients, while whole grains are so good for you, you can put something unhealthy with them and still reserve the right to feel like you're eating healthy. Vegetables and whole grains are good for you! Think of it this way—which is worse, having to choke down some vegetables every now and again or going on for months about how ethical, earth-friendly, and yummy veganism is, only to go to the doctor and find out (and have to tell everyone) that you're deficient in everything? Trust me, you will learn to like veggies eventually. Maybe you've just been eating them the wrong way—has a certain vegetable always been on your family's table mushy, oversalted, brown, or drowning in cheese? Just try preparing it a different way. For example, I usually dislike carrots when they're by themselves or mushy from being cooked, but I love dipping them, raw, in hummus. I'm not at all a fan of raw broccoli, but I love it when it's cooked. Likewise, have you only had spinach when it's squishy, dead, salted, and drowning in its own juices? That is *not* how spinach is meant to be—try some fresh and raw with pasta or in a wrap. The texture is semicrisp, not mushy, and the flavor isn't overpowering or bad. Even if you kinda like the way you're used to having a certain vegetable, you might like it just as much or even more in another way. Potatoes are great baked, fried, or mashed, sure, but they're also spectacular when you roast them with some olive oil, salt, pepper, and rosemary. There's always sneaking vegetables into foods if you know you need them but still don't like them, too. Make a pot of vegan mac 'n' cheeze and add tiny pieces of cooked broccoli to it. Sneak greens into a smoothie (aside from not being the best color, it tastes fine!). Hide corn and cut-up peppers in a bean burrito. When you eat a balanced, healthy diet, you can definitely go for that cone of vegan ice cream every now and then. If you really don't want to try to eat healthy, at least look at the next section.

SUPPLEMENTS

A supplement is a good idea whether you're a junk food vegan or not. Even if you're eating plenty of fruit, vegetables, and whole grains, taking a supplement is still smart. It's best to get vitamins and minerals from real food, but, just to be safe, round out your healthy diet with a daily multivitamin—this is something both vegans and omnivores alike should do. Besides, in certain cases, an artificial supplement might be your main source of a nutrient, like with vitamin B12. And if your real diet is heavy on the vegan nachos and sugary cereal, definitely take a multivitamin unless you feel like telling all your friends, teachers, and relatives that you went vegan and became deficient in calcium, iron, and whatever other nutrients you can think of. But will just any multivitamin do? Nope! first, you're a growing teenager, and second, you're vegan. Not all multivitamins are vegan—some contain gelatin and might contain vitamins that are derived from an animal product. You can buy vegan vitamins from vegan stores online (see page 143) or at health food stores, but if you go the second route, make sure it says *vegan* on the label. Some vitamins say "vegetarian" or "vegetarian formula" on the label, and this usually means that the supplement isn't made with gelatin, but it could still contain vitamins or other ingredients that are not from plant sources. I take VegLife brand Vegan Iron—it's available online or in any health food store, and has iron and B12 plus a little vitamin C and folic acid. The Whole Foods store brand also makes— get this—a vegan gummy vitamin. There are certain vitamins that need special attention during adolescence, particularly if you're female. Teenage girls need to make extra-certain that they're getting enough iron, and all teenagers need more calcium than adults do.

BUT MY DOCTOR SAYS...

Depending on things, your doctor may or may not think that it's healthy that you're vegan. Oftentimes parents— and almost everyone else for that matter—think that a doctor has the final authority on all issues concerning the body. Well, guess what—he/she doesn't. Doctors are not nutritionists or dieticians. In the United States, doctors usually take only one course on nutrition, ergo, they know about the same amount about nutrition as the average American...and the average American thinks that meat, dairy, and eggs are necessary for health. Doctors are trained to treat problems after they happen, not prevent them. If you want some medication for that particularly nasty flu, your doctor knows what to do. If you want to eat the healthiest diet you can, not to mention stave off the heart disease, cancer, osteoporosis, and other health issues that are becoming increasingly normal, your doctor does not really know what to do. So, take everything he or she tells you with a grain of salt—and all the books on vegan health you can find (see page 78), and the knowledge that the USDA food pyramid does in fact support vegan diets.

Chapter Five: Who's Who and What's What

★

Now that you're vegan, there are some things you have to know so that you're not laughed out of the next potluck you'll go to. Just kidding, vegans are a friendly bunch, but there are some things that would behoove you to learn as a new vegan. Want to know more about animal rights? Need to stock your shelves with good vegan cookbooks? Here ya go!

Books on Animal Rights

Slaughterhouse: The Shocking Story of Greed, Neglect, and Inhumane Treatment Inside the U.S. Meat Industry by Gail A. Eisnitz. This book delves into the world of factory-farming with an emphasis on human costs, such as working conditions on killing floors and the horrors of E. coli infections. If you want to know more about why factory farms are awful but are tired of hearing about battery cages and bolt guns, this is the book for you.

Empty Cages: Facing the Challenge of Animal Rights by Tom Regan. The title of this book comes from the credo of the abolitionist movement—we don't want bigger cages, we want empty cages. This book argues why we need to give all animals—whether human, dog, or other—the same moral consideration as we are all sentient beings and we all want to stay alive.

Eternal Treblinka: Our Treatment of Animals and the Holocaust by Marjorie Spiegel. This book makes the case for the comparison between the Holocaust and our treatment of animals now. Before your alarms start going off, know that the book has an entire section in which Holocaust survivors write on why they see their past experiences as connected to the experiences of animals today.

The Dreaded Comparison: Human and Animal Slavery by Marjorie Spiegel. Similar to Spiegel's above book, *The Dreaded Comparison* makes the connection between human treatment of other animals and white treatment of other humans. Rather than claim that these two forms of oppression are identical, she focuses on the chilling similarities between the relationship of oppressor and oppressed in both cases.

The Sexual Politics of Meat by Carol J. Adams. Ever wondered why male vegetarians are seen as effeminate or why ads for meat products so often feature animals that look like they want to be eaten? Read this. This is *the* book making the case for the connection between exploitation of women and of animals. A must-read for any feminist vegan.

Mad Cowboy by Howard Lyman. A bit of every major aspect of veganism from a cattle rancher turned vegan.

Meat Market by Erik Marcus. This is where you want to go for the real facts about what goes on within factory-farm walls, and, more importantly, why. Marcus doesn't appeal to sentimentality but rather states why the conditions in factory farms make economic sense, using agricultural journals and other sources from "the other side."

The Case for Animal Rights by Tom Regan. This is the seminal work on animal rights. Regan argues for abolitionist animal rights beautifully.

Introduction to Animal Rights: Your Child or the Dog? by Gary Francione. A great introduction to abolitionist animal rights if you've never read anything like this before.

Rain Without Thunder: The Ideology of The Animal Rights Movement by Gary Francione. This would be good after you've read more about animal rights, but it's a compelling read. Francione analyzes the two branches of the animal rights movement—abolitionism and welfare. He dismantles all the logic of welfarism. Yeah!

Books on Veganism in General

The Vegan Sourcebook by Joanne Stepaniak. One of the most engaging and multifaceted guides to veganism out there. In addition to the basic health info, history, and advice, you also get environmental info, great recipes, a sociological and psychological look at veganism, menu plans, and a list of other vegan resources and organizations.

Vegan: The New Ethics of Eating by Erik Marcus. A general guide to the ethical, health, and environmental reasons for being vegan. This highly informative book is also available for free download from vegan.com, the author's website.

Vegan Freak: Being Vegan in a Non-Vegan World by Bob and Jenna Torres. An everything guide to being vegan—great for new vegans! *Vegan Freak* is a great primer and provides the basics on health, social situations, food, ethics, and more.

Being Vegan by Joanne Stepaniak. One of the most definitive guides to being vegan. Practical, engaging information about the vegan philosophy and its usage in everyday life, food, the history of veganism, and more.

Cookbooks

Vegan with a Vengeance by Isa Chandra Moskowitz. Simply kick-ass. If you didn't get this at vegan orientation, there may have been an error processing your conversion. Tempeh bacon, Fauxstess cupcakes, jerk seitan, scones...*drool* Isa is half of the team behind *The Post Punk Kitchen*, a vegan cooking show on NYC public access.

How It All Vegan by Sarah Kramer and Tanya Barnard. The first in a great trilogy (but we're all crossing our fingers for it to be a tetralogy) of vegan cookbooks. Lots of delicious recipes for vegan basics. P.S. If you keep saying the title over and over again to yourself, make vegan rhyme with "began."

The Garden of Vegan by Sarah Kramer and Tanya Barnard. More from the Kramer & Barnard team, with a special section on microwave cooking, perfect for those of you in college or lazy like me!

La Dolce Vegan! by Sarah Kramer. Recipes from Sarah, recipes from fans, recipes for punk-as-fork crafts and earth-friendly cleaners, what's not to love? I might point you to the cinnamon doughnut holes or the roasted red pepper pesto. Most of these recipes are on the quick side (and they're all fantastic).

Vegan Cupcakes Take Over the World by Isa Chandra Moskowitz and Terry Hope Romero. Oh yeah, you read that title right. Banana split, s'mores, tiramisu, black forest, chocolate peanut butter...vegan cupcakes are most definitely going to take over the world. If you're ready to become a Certified Cupcake Hipster and see a dramatic increase in the number of friends you have as well as the size of the pants you wear, rejoice!

Vegan Cookies Invade Your Cookie Jar by Isa Chandra Moskowitz and Terry Hope Romero. The onslaught of vegan baked goods is endless from these two. In addition to all the basics, this cookbook features veganized versions of classics like Milano cookies and black-and-whites, plus bars, brownies, and everything from Sell Your Soul Pumpkin Cookies to Sweet Wine Biscuits with Sesame. Fancy!

Alternative Vegan by Dino Sarma. Now, I'll confess, I love a good omni-sub, but vegetables and spices are beautiful things. Behold a cookbook free of soymilk, tofu, tempeh, and all that other stuff—just wonderful, natural, delicious things ready to be tweaked to your own tastes.

The Native Foods Cookbook by Tanya Petrovna. Petrovna is the founder and owner of the Native Foods restaurants in southern California. These recipes are fresh and hella good. I'm a big fan of the Chinese Save-the-Chicken Salad and I've yet to find a better recipe for vegan ranch than in this book.

The Student's Go Vegan Cookbook by Carole Raymond. Pretty quick, pretty cheap, pretty easy—very delicious! A must for anyone in college. My favorite meal comes from this cookbook, Seitan Sauté with Pineapple.

The Student's Vegetarian Cookbook by Carole Raymond. Many vegan and easily veganized recipes for the broke, rushed, hungry vegan you are.

The Ultimate Uncheese Cookbook by Jo Stepaniak. Completely dairy-free recipes for vegan ricotta, feta, cheese sauce, cheezy spread, and more. And you thought you couldn't kick the habit.

Vegan Planet by Robin Robertson. One of the largest vegan cookbooks out there, *Vegan Planet* hits all the bases—ethnic foods, vegan versions of familiar foods, desserts, salads, sauces, and more.

The Everyday Vegan by Dreena Burton. A wide collection of easy-to-follow recipes for day-to-day vegan eating, as well as tips on nutrition, meal planning, and more.

Sinfully Vegan by Lois Dieterly. Desserts, desserts, and more desserts. Oh yeah. This is what you whip out when people tell you that vegan desserts are cardboard because chocolate caramel Boston cream pie, Death-by-Chocolate brownies, and creamy rice pudding don't sound like boxing material to me. Plus, *Sinfully Vegan* has over fifty wheat-free desserts, great if you are or know someone who is gluten intolerant.

Vive Le Vegan! by Dreena Burton. Similar to *The Everyday Vegan*, with more of an emphasis on family-friendly (read: quick and easy) recipes.

Vegan Lunch Box by Jennifer McCann. So maybe your mom doesn't pack you utterly amazing vegan lunches, but you can pretend. How lucky would you be to open up your lunchbox and find potstickers, a vegan Twinkie, mini vegan pizzas, or roasted tomato basil soup? Almost makes you want to go to school...

Veganomicon by Isa Chandra Moskowitz and Terry Hope Romero. The bible of vegan cooking, the ultimate vegan cookbook, a never-ending tome of delicious recipes and good information. From basic cooking skills to fancy complicated recipes, this one goes all out.

Books on Health

The China Study by T. Colin Campbell. If you read just one book on vegan health, this is it. The fact that it isn't written by an animal-rights guy is a great fact to throw at incredulous omnis. The argument against diets with animal products is never clearer or more convincing than in *The China Study*. Some of the results of his studies simply blew me away. It gives a new meaning to the phrase "go vegan or die."

Diet for A New America by John Robbins. This is one of the first books on veg*nism for health and a great source for the basics. Robbins was the heir to the Baskin-Robbins ice cream fortune but decided being vegan was more fun.

Becoming Vegan: The Complete Guide to Adopting a Healthy Plant-Based Diet by Brenda Davis. Rather than focus on the negative effects of not being vegan, this book is a guide to what you need to do to be a healthy vegan with a healthy diet. Read it! Eat your veggies!

The Vegan Sourcebook by Joanne Stepaniak. A general guide to being an herbivore, with some great basic information about vegan health and nutrition.

Animal-Related Organizations

Vegan Outreach makes those lovely little *Why Vegan?* pamphlets that you've probably seen, among several others, like a great *Guide to Cruelty-Free Eating* with recipes, nutritional info, and more. While some people don't like that they're not explicitly abolitionist, their overall message is to go vegan, and that's what matters. Website: www.veganoutreach.org

Action for Animals provides a great vegan starter kit and does a lot of the tabling you may have seen at big concerts like the Warped tour. Website: www.afa-online.org

Compassion Over Killing is responsible for a wide variety of campaigns, including the abolition of the "Animal Care Certified" label on egg cartons. They also provide material for library displays, veggie starter guides, leaflets, and more. Website: www.cok.net

People for the Ethical Treatment of Animals is the oldest and best-known animal rights organization in the world. While they are known as the most extreme of the extremists, they're actually quite moderate and welfarist. PETA runs GoVeg.com, VegCooking.com, and a slew of related websites. Website: www.peta.org

In Defense of Animals operates animal sanctuaries in Mississippi and in Africa, in addition to holding educational events, providing resources for grassroots activism, and much more. Website: www.idausa.org

The Animal Liberation Front isn't really an organization because they're not particularly organized. Rather, "Any group of people who are vegetarians or vegans and who carry out actions according to ALF guidelines have the right to regard themselves as part of the ALF." The ALF is mainly known for its love of direct action (rescuing animals and causing financial loss to animal exploiters). Website: www.animalliberationfront.com

Farm Sanctuary is mainly known for its work rescuing animals and its farm sanctuaries in California and in New York State, but they also work for policy reform and animal welfare campaigns. Website: www.farmsanctuary.org

Peaceful Prairie is the only abolitionist farm sanctuary out there. PP operates in Colorado and is home to several incredibly lucky pigs, sheep, chickens, cows, geese, and other animals. Website: www.peacefulprairie.org

Friends of Animals is an international animal advocacy organization based in Connecticut. They work for a wide variety of campaigns, including spaying/neutering programs, protecting the rights of free-living (wild) animals, and providing disaster/emergency relief for animals. Website: www.friendsofanimals.org

Chapter Six: Vegan Goodies

I have a secret for you. Vegans eat cookies. Vegans wear belts. Vegans use shampoo. Going vegan means giving up animal products, but not products themselves! There are great vegan alternatives to things you probably used/consumed a lot when you weren't vegan. You can be a vegan and still eat ice cream sandwiches, sprinkle parmesan on your pasta, put on lip balm when your lips are dry, pour milk on your cereal, wear makeup, eat candy, wash your hands, and virtually everything else you used to do from before you were vegan—simply use vegan alternatives to traditionally non-vegan items. This chapter is mainly a guide to the products themselves; for places to buy a lot of this stuff online, see Chapter 12.

Body Products

The task of finding toiletries that contain no animal products and are not tested on animals may seem daunting at first. After all, many items (such as glycerin) can be derived from both plants and animals, and labels don't often specify where such ingredients came from. Many products use sneaky labeling—when it says "This finished product is not tested on animals," it means that while the final, complete product isn't tested on animals, its ingredients still could be. What's a vegan to do? Washing your hair is pretty much necessary. Hands get dry and need lotion. Putting on makeup sometimes is fun. You can't just not use things and you really don't want to support (read: buy) products that aren't vegan. Well, like most aspects of veganism, after a while, finding vegan body products isn't so hard. You learn which brands to use and which to avoid. You figure out where to get them. What kind of person uses more body products than the average teenage girl? Well, I'm a teenage girl, and I'm a vegan. Once I was a new vegan and the idea of jumping through hoops just to find out if I wanted to buy a certain brand of lip balm wasn't so appealing to me. Now, though, I have a bathroom filled with body products and they're all vegan. I've never jumped through any hoops. I've just learned over the time I've been vegan which brands of things are vegan and which are not. Here I've gathered some of these brands so that you, too, can smell nice, be moisturized, and all that other stuff—while still being the vegan that you are!

Rather than name all the specific animal ingredients, I'm going to tell you what has been easier for and more helpful to me than memorizing lists of ingredients: knowing which roots of words mean animal products. Online, you can find lists of all the ingredients that may be derived from animals, and while I do recommend you do this, I recommend this only to familiarize yourself with these ingredients. Very few people can keep extensive lists of weird-sounding ingredients constantly in their minds, and I'm not one of them. Plus, since there are many individual ingredients that are merely different forms of each other, remembering one three- or four-letter root is simply much easier than trying to remember a handful of related ingredients, and it was just what naturally happened for me when I was phasing out and replacing my non-vegan toiletries. Knowing the roots of animal products also helps you decide whether an ingredient you've never seen is derived from animals or not.

These ingredients are yummy and you definitely want to be smearing them all over your body. Animal ingredients in toiletries, cosmetics, perfumes, and other body products are obtained in some nasty ways. The juices of crushed bugs (carmine), fatty intestinal buildup from whales (ambergris), urine (cystine, among others), blood and muscle tissue (lactic acid), and similar parts of beings find their way into a wide variety of body products. Deeee-licious.

Lac	(like lactose and lactic acid).
Lan	(like lanolin and lanogene).
Stear	(like calcium stearate and stearic acid).
Ur	(like uric acid and urea).
Al	(like albumen and aldioxa).
Ine	(means it's an amino acid, which are commonly derived from animals. For example, alanine and cysteine.)
Estr	(like estrogen and estradiol).
Lip	(like lipids and lipase)
Tallow	(like tallow acid and tallow amine)

Was that difficult? Online, you can find lists of all the ingredients that may be derived from animals, and while I do recommend you do this, I recommend this only to familiarize yourself with these ingredients. Remembering the roots is just much easier. And let's face it, once you know a few things, veganism's pretty easy. And now here they are, the brands. Vegan body products will be yours! Again, these products are usually available in health food stores, always available online, and sometimes available in average places where you least expect them.

Aveda is almost an entirely vegan company. None of its products are tested on animals, and aside from beeswax/honey in certain products, they're almost all vegan. Makeup, shampoo, conditioner, skin-care products, hair products, and more. They're a little on the costly side, but they're very good quality. Plus, Aveda also has salons/spas, so they're a great place to go if you feel like getting a pedicure or something and want it done without the worry of animal testing. You can buy their products at their website or in their stores. Website: www.aveda.com

Kiss My Face is also almost entirely vegan. None of its products are tested on animals, and only a few of them contain insect-derived ingredients. Kiss My Face makes shower gel, hand soap, deodorant, lip balm, and more. You can buy their products at most health food stores and on their website. KMF also makes a line of products for Old Navy stores that are also mostly vegan. Website: www.kissmyface.com

J/A/S/O/N is a completely vegan company. They use strictly plant ingredients in its products, which are even certified as not tested on animals. Jason makes toothpaste, deodorant, hair-care products, hand soap, face washes and scrubs, mouthwash, and more. You can buy their products at most health food stores and on their website. Website: www.jason-natural.com

Method is a completely vegan company that makes household products (like cleaning supplies, air freshener, and the like) in addition to some body products. While its range of body products is not as extensive as that of other companies, you can still buy hand soap, body wash, and hand sanitizers from them, either from their website or at most major chains. Website: www.methodhome.com

Tom's of Maine is also a completely vegan company. They are mainly known for their oral-care products like toothpaste and mouthwash, but they also sell deodorant, skin-care products, soap, and more. Their products are available everywhere from healthfood stores to major chains. Website: www.tomsofmaine.com

The Merry Hempsters do not test their products on animals but use insect-derived ingredients in certain items. However, they do sell vegan lip balm, salve, lotion, and more—their vegan products even say vegan right in the name! You can buy their products on their website and in most healthfood stores and head shops. Website: www.merryhempsters.com

Lush is a U.K-based company that does not test any of its products on animals and uses animal ingredients in only a few of its items. They make amazingly yummy soaps, bath bombs, hair-care products, lip balm, perfume, shaving cream, and much more. Unless you live in the U.K., your only option is to buy their products from their website, which clearly specifies which products are vegan and which aren't. Website: www.lush.com

Alba does not test any of its products on animals. Their ingredients tend to be vegan, but a few products contain ingredients like honey and lanolin. They make a wide range of products, from skin-care to hair-care to deodorant and lip balm. You can buy their products at most healthfood stores or on their website. Website: www.albabotanica.com

Nature's Gate is a completely vegan company. They make hair-care products, skin-care, lip balm, fragrances, deodorant, sunscreen, and much more. You can buy their products at most-health food stores or on their website. Website: www.natures-gate.com

Freeman is another completely vegan company. They make skin-care products, body wash/shower gel, lotion, hand and foot care products, hair-care products, and more. Unlike most of the other companies I've listed, they are available not in healthfood stores but in many mainstream stores (as well as online). Website: www.freemanbeauty.com

Yes To branches off into three different lines—Yes To Carrots, Cucumbers, and Tomatoes. Basically, each line is for a different kind of skin or hair (normal, dry, or oily, respectively), and none of their products are tested on animals. Some contain honey, so read the label, but that's the only animal ingredient they use. Their stuff smells great and lasts a long time.

Giovanni makes slightly higher-end hair-care products that are all organic and vegan. I particularly like their Frizz Be Gone smoothing serum. A little goes a long way and it makes you smell like you live your life in a fancy salon.

These are just some of the many vegan body product companies (and non-vegan companies with vegan products, like L'Oreal's EverPure line) out there. Poke around your local healthfood store or even your local beauty supply store—you'll never know what's vegan unless you look!

Food

There are great-tasting, nutritious (and sometimes not-so-nutritious) alternatives to pretty much any non-vegan food you can dream up. Don't be afraid of your local healthfood store, because you'll probably be surprised at the wide variety of vegan product options it carries. Whether it's chicken nuggets, coffee creamer, frozen pizza, whipped butter, ice cream bars, mayonnaise, cheese puffs, beef crumbles, honey, yogurt smoothies, pudding cups, cheese slices, lunchmeat, or whatever else you're missing, there are vegan versions out there that look and taste the same. I've even eaten mock snails before (they were actually quite tasty) and seen vegan haggis online. Speaking of online, if you live in a small town and don't have a healthfood store or it's just really small and pathetic, you can order a lot of these alternatives online (see page 143). But you don't even have to have a healthfood store in a lot of cases! Never in my life (well, never in my life when I was paying attention) did I go to a grocery store that didn't have a healthfood *section* at the very least which carried the essentials. Even the average chain groceries in my city carry fake meat and vegan ice cream. The mom-and-pop grocery store you've been going to all your life may have awesome vegan products hidden away that you simply don't know about because you've never looked! If you're looking for names of specific brands, VegProductsGuide.com is a great place to start. Also, you may be surprised how many foods you're used to eating are "accidentally vegan." Many popular brands of crackers, cereals, cookies, and the like are vegan without really intending to be. When I became vegan, even though I did (and still do) love a good omni-sub, I grew to like vegetables, grains, fruits, and legumes by themselves, when they weren't imitating anything. Vegan food is easy to find!

Clothes

Going through your closet, you may find that a lot of products like belts and shoes are made of leather, or that your winter coat is made of wool or stuffed with down. Before you decide that your possession of these items means you aren't and can never be vegan, know that there are vegan alternatives (surprise surprise!) out there. Also, the vegan police are *not* going to chase you down and arrest you for still having animal products in your clothing. Very few people can afford to throw out all their non-vegan shoes, belts, coats, jackets, purses, shirts, skirts, and so forth and buy completely new ones. Most people just don't have money like that. Nobody is going to blame you for wearing down your leather shoes until they're falling apart or for veganizing your wardrobe bit by bit rather than all at once. Though, please, if you're going out to leaflet or something, leave the leather jacket at home. A lot of people assume that if you're wearing leather you support the industry itself and continue to buy animal products, and then think you're a hypocrite if you're trying to change people's minds about veganism. If you're not leafleting/protesting, but can't afford to replace your wool coat and people know you're vegan, simply explain that veganism is about eliminating animal products as much as is possible/practical, and right now it's neither possible nor practical for you to splurge on a new vegan coat.

When you are ready to replace your leather belts with pleather ones and your silk pajamas with satin ones, you have (like with everything else, no?) plenty of options. Many vegan websites (see page 143) sell vegan alternatives to non-vegan clothing, but there's stuff in the real world, too. Many less-expensive shoe stores, like Payless, use pleather in their shoes. You can find cloth or vegan fleece jackets at many stores, cotton sweaters if you look hard enough (thrift stores are your friend!), and pleather belts at a wide variety of stores.

While some people may say that it's technically vegan to buy leather, wool, etc. secondhand, I don't think it is. Although you do not support these industries directly if you buy their products from thrift stores, you still support the idea that animals are ours to wear, and that ain't cool.

Chapter Seven: Outreach, School, Etc.

★

Now probably more than any of the other time you're going to be vegan, you have the most potential for activism. I mean this both in the sense that you're young and have more energy and free time than you would if you were older, and that you've just gone vegan and all the knowledge of more people need to be vegan is fresh in your mind and heart. Everything feels new and exciting. You want to change minds. You want to change lives! And that's a great feeling, no matter how long you've been vegan.

While the most obvious form of activism, protesting, is great, you might not be the protesting type, your parents might think that's too drastic, or you simply might be the only vegan (that you know of) in your area. Protesting is just fine, but it is definitely not the only form of activism there is—in most cases, protesting isn't the most effective way of getting the message out there. It takes a lot of different tactics to effect change and sometimes standing outside of a building with a sign in your hand and a scream in your throat doesn't do much more than release some of your anger. There are plenty of simple, effective ways of changing minds that don't require a megaphone, and there are plenty of things you can do if your parents are like mine used to be—comfortable with me being vegan, but not so turned on to the idea of me trying to spread my beliefs.

The bottom line is that veganism alone is a start. While it is necessary, yes, and while veganism does shape the way you think about things and see the world, the simple act of not consuming certain things is not the end. How would anybody go vegan if nobody made any effort about outreach? Somebody had to make that video you saw. Somebody had to write that book you read. Somebody had to talk to you. Somebody sat in front of a computer making that website you checked out, somebody handed you that leaflet... If everyone who went vegan just holed themselves up and never made any attempt to change things, well, things simply would not change.

You don't have to be great at giving speeches and you don't have to live in a city where there's a protest every weekend. I like to write, so I wrote a book about being a teenage vegan. The overlap between the vegan and nerd communities is strong, which explains why there are a lot of websites and Internet-related projects related to veganism (though you don't have to be a nerd to set up a simple blog.) A friend of mine is a teacher, so he teaches a class about animal rights. Many artists use their art to say something about animal rights. Everybody has something they're good at and more often than not you can use your talent to do some really great activism. Now get out there and change some minds!

Leafleting can be a really effective, easy way to work for positive change, and it's especially fun if you recruit a few friends to help you out. find a time and place where a lot of people are walking around, get a stack of pamphlets, and get to it! Smile and look pleasant when you hand them out—not like you're there against your will or like veganism has sucked the joy from your life. My vegan friends and I leaflet when the galleries in the local art district put out new stuff and everyone goes down to take a look. Pamphlets are available from Vegan Outreach (www.veganoutreach.org) and are usually at a discount to vegan groups (?). It's also fun, albeit a little more effort, to print up your own little zine about veganism, or maybe just about your local veg*n scene—is there a meetup or other event coming up? Did a restaurant just add some exciting vegan dishes to its menu? When you do leaflet, make sure you're prepared to answer any and all questions people have, as well as deal with the hilarious and unique individuals who have nothing better to do with their lives than tell you about the great slab of steak they just polished off. If you hand out a mere hundred pamphlets in one go, and if only 1 percent (a very conservative estimate) of the people to whom you hand leaflets makes the decision to go vegan, vegetarian, or just reduce the amount of animal products they consume, that's still one entire life changed and countless animals saved from being born into a factory farm.

Leaving leaflets is also good if you don't have the time to stand around and talk to people or it would be a weird place to. Coffee shops and libraries are good places to start. Talk to the owners of coffee shops and see if they'll let you leave a stack of pamphlets every so often. My local vegan group has most of the independent coffee shops in the area "adopted"— somebody nearby drops off a stack of leaflets every weekend or so, and every leaflet gets taken! I mean, you're there for coffee/tea/socialization anyway, right, so why not get some positive social change with your cup of joe? Libraries typically have other information and leaflets from various groups out, so why not ask the librarian if you can leave leaflets. Another sneaky tactic my friends and I have used is commandeering those stands you see on street corners. You know, the ones that usually have information about buying houses and whatnot. Nobody was really using them so they just started leaving *Why Vegan?*s in them. Of course, eventually the city realized what was going on and took the stands away, but nobody got in trouble...

Even having leaflets on you is great. At school, I have a *Why Vegan?* and a *Guide to Cruelty-Free Eating* in the folder I take to all my classes. With the pocket of the folder, you can just see the title of the first booklet. This alone is often intriguing enough to my classmates for them to ask if they can see it! Plus, when you're a new vegan, you may not yet feel entirely comfortable talking about the issues with people. When I had just gone vegan, I usually felt like the leaflet would do a better job of explaining things than I would, and simply gave people a sentence or two and a leaflet when they asked me about my veganism. Now I'm generally comfortable enough to actually talk to people about veganism, but it took time, and the leaflets were a big help.

Being a good example is constant activism! It's also, in my opinion, what gets the most people to go vegan. Even if someone is faced with the grim reality of factory farming, they're probably not going to make much of a change if they have the idea that all vegans are crusty hippies with bland, repetitive diets who are lightning-quick to loudly chastise someone who eats whey. We're not all like that, and, in fact, very few us are. What if a person found out about factory farming and thought of the real live vegan they knew? That real live vegan who is just as healthy as anyone else, makes great food, has a life, doesn't cut herself off from her friends even when she disagrees with them? Then that person would know that being veganism is not only possible, but tasty, pretty easy, and all that other good stuff. It opens someone's mind incredibly when you defy the negative stereotype most people have of vegans. Make an effort to show people that you don't eat an exclusive diet of lettuce and cardboard and try your best to be calm and approachable rather than angry and shut-off about your veganism.

Culinary activism is like being a good example and just as important. People have the misconception that vegan food is tasteless and that vegan desserts are bland and dry. If you've ever had a plate of Thai peanut noodles, a bowl of creamy dairy-free chocolate pudding, a slice of field roast with veggie gravy, and so many other delicious vegan things, you know this isn't true! Oftentimes, the true flavors of a food come out even stronger when they aren't overpowered with dead animal. And oftentimes the people who have such a bad impression of what vegan food is haven't really had any! Whether you have a friend over and make them your favorite meal, bring cupcakes to a friend's party, or just pack things other than peanut butter and jelly for lunch (see page 114), you can show the people in your life that going vegan does not mean giving up flavor, diversity, or the enjoyment of food. I have had great success with culinary activism in the past.

I throw parties a lot for my friends, and I like doing this. Whenever I do, I always put out a nice blend of vegan versions of omni foods and delicious things my friends have never eaten. Now, my friends are always more excited about the parties I throw than the ones our other friends do, because they know I have better food! At another friend's house, it'll be chips and dip, maybe some candy. At my house, it'll be hummus and pita chips, some accidentally vegan candy, a frozen cheeseless pizza, vegan onion dip in a bread bowl, cookies...whatever!

Once I was spending the night at an omni friend's house, and we wanted to make cookies. I was able to find a recipe that didn't call for soymilk or egg replacer or anything, and they turned out wonderfully. Her parents even commented that they tasted better than "normal" oatmeal cookies.

In French class, we had a party. I brought some chocolate cupcakes that went over wonderfully, but there were some extras. My next class was small, so I thought I would share the leftover cupcakes with them. Everyone loved them, and one of my friends—a hardcore omni who remarked that vegan cupcakes "taste like poo" before he tried one—went back for a second one.

During my sophomore year of high school, everyone in the group I ate with brought their lunch. My omni friends usually brought peanut butter and jelly, a bologna sandwich, or something like that. The lunches I brought were so good that it wasn't at all uncommon for me to simply say "I have a good lunch today!" and then for them to start guessing what it was and suggesting yummy things I had brought in the past. One day, one of my friends turned to me and made a comment about how it was funny—my diet is the most restricted, but my lunches are the best-tasting, best-smelling, and most creative.

But it's no wonder—you don't need eggs to bind things together. You don't need milk to make something creamy. You don't need meat to make something hearty and filling. Vegan food tastes good!

Be a walking billboard and wear clothing with a vegan message. If you're going to walk around all day advertising something on your chest, why not make it be veganism, rather than whatever corporation or clothing store can get you to wear their logo? Wearing something that promotes veganism is a great way for another person to start a conversation with you about it, for restaurants to see that they have vegan customers, and for everyone to see that there are real vegans in their city, workplace, or school. What you wear doesn't have to be confrontational—there are plenty of tees, tanks, hoodies, and sweatshirts out there with messages that are friendly *and* vegan. For a list of online stores where you can buy these items, see page 143.

Opportunities in school are chances for activism that are unique to being a teen vegan. Most adults don't get to write papers about veganism or give presentations on animal rights for work, but you might get to! Assignments where you get to the pick the topic are common. Not only is a subject to do with veganism more interesting to you (meaning you'll probably work harder at it and get a better grade), but it's awesome vegan outreach.

During my freshman year of high school, my English class had to write a research paper on the topic of our choice, and I wrote about the health benefits of a vegan diet as compared to a vegetarian or omnivorous one. I had a blast getting to spend weeks and weeks of school time learning about veganism, and what I learned amazed me. I was only five or six months into being vegan, and I think that learning so much about how wise it is to be vegan was a big help. My paper got one of the highest grades in the class, and I had lots of fun writing it.

At the end of that same year, my final for one of my classes was a presentation on whatever I wanted, and I picked veganism. I did a little bit on the ethical, health, and environmental reasons to be vegan, and some FAQs omnis have about veganism, like what I eat and where I get certain nutrients. It went wonderfully and I was really pleased to have an opportunity to talk about veganism with my classmates.

You can probably work veganism into any project involving:

Social movements. Although vegetarianism has been a movement for many centuries, veganism has really taken off in the Western world in the past few decades, and the number of vegans is increasing. You could talk about the evolution of the movement, the different submovements within it (like welfarists, abolitionists, health vegans, etc.), the movement's future, the increasing availability of vegan products in mainstream stores, or more.

Food. Vegan food is definitely different from the meat-and-potatoes that most Americans are used to. You could talk about some of your favorite vegan meals, types of ethnic cuisine that shy away from animal products (like Indian, Japanese, or Mediterranean, to name a few), common vegan foods, or more. Make this project more exciting by preparing some vegan food and sharing it with your teacher and class!

Philosophy. If your personal philosophy involves equality and nonviolence, you're not alone. Notable veg*n thinkers/philosophers include: Henry David Thoreau,

Mahatma Gandhi, George Bernard Shaw, Albert Einstein, Leonardo da Vinci, Franz Kafka, Leo Tolstoy, Plato, and more. Another great resource is Vegan Outreach's page on veganism and philosophy, located at www.veganoutreach.org/advocacy/beyond.html.

Health. Like I've said before, the vegan diet can be the healthiest one there is, and vegetarianism and omnivorism tend to be nutritional train wrecks. Turn to page 78 for a list of books about veganism and health.

Oppression. Most people would think of women or minorities if they were asked for an oppressed group. However, few people would think of animals even though the comparisons between the three groups are numerous.

Destruction of the environment. Fun fact: switching from the standard American diet to a vegan one saves more fossil fuel per year than switching from a regular car to a Prius. Animal agriculture gobbles up resources and contributes greatly to pollution, as well as being a less efficient way to transfer energy than eating plant foods directly.

and whatever else you can think of!

Starting a veg*n club. This is more work than other things, but if you've got a decent veg community at your school (or even if you don't, and you want to change this) go for it! find out what your school's policy for starting a club is—most need a teacher to make sure you aren't planning to blow up the school or anything like that.

Once you've got the green light from the administration, set the date of your first meeting with enough time to gather interest. Tell all your veg friends or veg*ns at your school about the club. Make flyers. Most schools will let you make an announcement about your club with the rest of the day's announcements. You might want to make your first meeting a big celebratory deal, you might not. Either way, make sure to have plenty of literature and information for people who want it, and food. People like food.

Once you get around to having regular meetings, you may want to have a set meeting agenda or you may not. It's perfectly fine just to put out some vegan cookies and a stack of leaflets and talk about whatever veg-related issues pop into your head. But you also might want to tackle projects, like making your cafeteria more veg-friendly or setting up a display in the library. It's your club, after all.

Bumper stickers are such an easy way of letting the world know that there are vegans out there. If you have your own car, slap a few on! You'll send a simple message every time you drive.

Ask for vegan food when you go places that are lacking in it. If you're continually disappointed that your favorite local coffee shop doesn't have any vegan baked goods, tell them that you'd like to see some! Requesting vegan menu items lets restaurants know that there is a demand for such items. If they don't notice a demand for animal-free foods, it's doubtful that they'll put any on the menu. On the other hand, if they *do* notice an increasing demand for vegan menu items, don't be surprised if there are suddenly a few good veg options on a formerly all-meat menu. Ask and ye shall receive.

Tabling is great at concerts, fairs, and other events. Most of the time you'll have to clear your table with somebody in charge of the event. Basically, get a table, stack it with literature and vegan treats and whatever else you can think of, and go to town. Hand out whatever you're handing out and be prepared to talk to people. Go for an area of the concert/fair with plenty of foot traffic and recruit a friend or two to help you. Some animal-related organizations (page 79) will give you free literature/posters/stickers/etc. if they know you're tabling, but remember that you're pimping veganism and not the organization itself. Keep your display friendly and inviting rather than gory and confrontational. Colors are good. Pictures of half-skinned pigs, not so much. Your table should look inviting. Although the cruel realities of animal agriculture are important to let people know about, people are far quicker to write off/ignore a gory, depressing message than a pleasant, inviting one. Make sure whatever literature you're handing out has adequate information should people want to learn even more about going veg.

Bake sales are awesome. Who doesn't love cookies and cupcakes? Stupid people, that's who. You'll probably have to clear this with your principal or another administrator before you get started, but beyond that, it's pretty simple. Secure a space—preferably one where lots of foot traffic will pass—and set up a table. Bake as many treats as you can (recruit your friends and their ovens if need be) and go for crowd-pleasers like snickerdoodles, brownies, cupcakes—you could even make a cake and sell the individual slices. Pimp the fact that the goodies are cholesterol-free, delicious, and, of course, free of animal products! You could even have a few pamphlets and other info about going veg on your table. Once the whole shebang is over, donate your earnings to a farm sanctuary (like Peaceful Prairie), Compassion Over Killing, or another animal rights organization (see page 79 for a full list).

Bottom line for activism: Be pleasant. Seem like a normal person who just happens to be vegan. Don't be confrontational. Do be informed. It's okay to accept that veganism is not the magical answer to everything. Don't expect everyone you meet to be all-ears to what you have to say, but also don't expect everyone to be idiotic and rude.

Burnout isn't going to get anyone to go vegan but it still belongs in this section. Avoiding burnout is important. It is so much better to do a manageable amount of outreach now and then for a long time than to go really hardcore for a short period of time and then give up forever. Nobody is perfect and nobody stays a hardcore activist for their entire life without negative effects. If you're constantly hearing animals scream in your head and being frustrated that you're doing so much but not seeing the level of change you would like, you need to step back and take a deep breath. Being an activist is different from driving yourself crazy with stress and frustration. If you start to feel like you're burning out, let up on some of your activism. Concentrate on the more fun parts of veganism, like trying new recipes and watching silly vegan videos like Steven the Vegan online. Go to potlucks rather than protests. Remind yourself why you're vegan and also remind yourself that you have your entire life to be an activist. Remember that you're not the only one working for change and the entire movement does not rest upon your shoulders. Remember that if you kill yourself overdoing activism now, you're not going to feel like doing any activism later. Calm down, relax, and when you're feeling back up to it, ease back into activism.

School-Related Ethical Conflicts

Dissection depends so much on your teacher. My biology teacher let anyone who wanted to do a virtual dissection instead of the real one and was generally very laid-back about the whole thing. Another teacher that many of my friends had refused to let the squeamish and vegetarian students do an alternative assignment. As soon you find out a dissection is scheduled, meet with your teacher before or after school as soon as you can. You may surprised how accommodating your teacher is—I was all ready to go and literally did not even get to finish my first sentence because she interrupted and assured me that I could do something else. Research the alternatives (like virtual ones—there are some online and many organizations will loan CD-ROMs and other programs for more in-depth virtual dissections) beforehand. Tell your teacher that you would like to perform one of these alternatives because dissection "violates your deeply held moral and religious beliefs." It's better to pretend for a day that you're a Jain or Buddhist than to have to do something you have deep ethical problems with, and it's often the word "religious" that gets teachers/administrators to take your concerns seriously. firmly establish with your teacher that you would be unsatisfied with just watching since that would be indirect participation, but participation nonetheless, in something you're against. Also firmly establish that you are willing to put out as much as effort in the alternative than you would in the actual dissection. If your teacher still ignores you, take it up with the principal—or, if he/she ignores you, the superintendent and school board. It's not as if the teacher is going to hold the scalpel in your hand and physically force you to dissect the frog, or whatever other animal it is. Remember to be calm and polite during all your interactions with your teacher. Start a petition among students if they still refuse to let you have an alternative—you're not going to be the only one in your school who isn't leaping for joy about the idea of cutting up an animal and poking at its organs. Happy virtual dissection!

Home Ec is a class that you should try and avoid if at all possible. I mean, I've never heard of a school that requires students to take it. But if you went vegan after you signed up for it, dropping the class might not be an option. Most schools let you drop a class the first week or so of taking it, but beyond that, even if you're now a passionate vegan, you've got to take what you signed up for. However, there is stuff you can do about it. Make sure your teacher knows what you do and do not eat. If you're cooking individually, see if he/she will allow you do a similar but alternative assignment. For example, when I was vegetarian (but not yet vegan) I was in a Home Ec–type class and we were supposed to make hamburgers. I made a meatless one at home, brought in a sample for the teacher, and still got full credit. If you're cooking in groups, try to get the jobs that involve dealing with the food as little as possible, like preheating the oven, handing utensils to the people actually cooking, drying dishes, and setting the table.

I've never heard of a teacher refusing to give points for not eating a dish, but if that happens, stress that eating whatever it is violates your deeply held ethical and moral principles. Use weighty phrases like that; it works out better than, "But I'm vegan."

A Bit About College

There are so many factors that go into choosing a college other than its level of vegan-friendliness, but it's something to think about. As a general rule of thumb, it seems like smaller liberal-arts schools tend to have more vegan options than larger state universities, but there are a lot of the latter that do plenty to keep their vegan students well-fed. Peta2 does publish a list every year of "America's Most Vegan-Friendly Colleges," but it's not an exhaustive one. I found it more informative to look at potential schools' websites—if you click around enough, most have their dining hall's weekly menu somewhere and it's easy to tell what it would be like to be a vegan there. My personal two cents: if you can make it to a school that takes care of its vegans, it does provide a nice foundation for increased day-to-day happiness. I went from taking my lunch every day in high school to Philly cheeze seitan subs and arugala explosions in college, and it admittedly rocks. But if cafeteria trips seem like they'll be the best thing about a school, it's not worth it, and if you go a school that isn't Veganopolis, that doesn't mean you'll be miserable. I have a vegan friend at a big state school that is a bit of a struggle for herbivorous scholars, but because she loves everything else about the school so much, she's made it work and is very happy. A word to the wise, no matter where you end up—hot pots and rice cookers are your best friends. They're small even by dorm standards, cheap, they plug in anywhere, and with enough creativity you can get them to make sooo many more things than the instruction manual says you should.

Chapter Eight: All the Rest

★

This chapter serves to gather together all the random (but still important) information you may like to know as a vegan, and even some fun and helpful things that even seasoned vegan teens may benefit from. Enjoy!

Bands with Vegan Members

I am definitely against going vegan just because the lead singer of your favorite band happens to be veg. Celebrity worship is bad. If you think that going vegan will mean you have even more in common with a certain famous person, not only is that the lamest of reasons for going vegan, but you're actually creating more reasons why you are different from this person. They're most likely vegan because of serious ethical, health, or environmental concerns, while you're vegan to be a groupie. Not cool. But let's put my cynicism aside, because I think only a very small percentage of people reading this are vegan for celebrity-worship reasons. It's just fun to know that members of your favorite bands are vegan like you—plus, vegan artists sometimes write songs about veganism or advocate for animals in other ways, which is cool. You might be surprised how many members of popular bands just say no to animal products!

* AFI (all members)
* Andy Hurley of Fall Out Boy
* Bill Hamilton of Silverstein
* Bill Ward of

Black Sabbath
* Brian Bell of Weezer
* Bryan Adams
* Bob Marley
* Cedric Bixer of the
  Mars Volta
* Chrissie Hynde of the
  Pretenders
* Common
* Dead Prez
* Dennis Lyxzen of the
  (International) Noise
  Conspiracy
* Erykah Badu
* Fiona Apple
* Forrest Kline of
  Hellogoodbye
* Fred Mascherino of
  Taking Back Sunday
* Geezer Butler of
  Black Sabbath
* Good Clean Fun (all
  members)
* I Object! (all members)
* Ian MacKaye of Minor
  Threat, Fugazi, etc.

* Johnny Whitney of
  Blood Brothers
* Mike Gordon of Phish
* Moby
* Morrissey
* Most Precious Blood
  (all members)
* Oi Polloi (all members)
* Omar Rodriguez-Lopez
  of the Mars Volta
* Paul McCartney
* Pink
* Prince
* Propagandhi (all
  members)
* Shane Told of
  Silverstein
* Shania Twain
* Sinead O'Connor
* Steve Jocz of Sum 41
* Ted Leo
* Thom Yorke of
  Radiohead
* Weird Al Yankovic
* Yoko Ono Lennon

Welfarism vs. Abolitionism

There are two branches of the animal rights movement, welfarism and abolitionism. Although these branches profess to have the same end goals, they are vastly different. A welfarist vegan and an abolitionist vegan, while both vegans, will find themselves butting heads all too often. So what's the difference?

Welfarists support free-range meat and cage-free eggs. They figure that since not everyone is going to go vegan, it's the least we can do to get them to choose "happy" meat. They also figure that animal exploitation isn't going to be over with anytime soon, and nothing we do can change that, so they spend their energy fighting for things like cage-free eggs and pigs who never see gestation crates. Through gradual increases in animal welfare legislation, they hope that humans will eventually come to see animals in a different light and stop exploiting them. For now, though, they're happy with bigger cages and quicker deaths. They think the end of animal exploitation will come, but not for a long, long time, and they don't think there's much they can do about this.

Abolitionists get their name from the abolitionist movement of the nineteenth century. Back then, abolitionists didn't want slave ships to be more comfortable or chains to be longer. They didn't waste their time compromising with slaveholders and asking them to please just whip a little more softly. They didn't tell plantation owners who really, really didn't want to give up their slaves to at least make sure their slaves were a little happier. They knew that humans were not property! Today, abolitionists are no different. Animals are not property, they're beings. We don't want bigger cages, we want empty cages. We don't want quicker slaughter, we want no slaughter. We want to work for abolitionism in our daily lives, and we know we can do it!

You've probably guessed by now that I'm an abolitionist. Yup. I have two main problems with welfarism: it accepts defeat before it even begins; and it asserts that animals are property. Welfarism assumes that not everyone can go vegan because nonwelfarist activism tactics are simply not effective enough. I admit, there are some people who are simply very unlikely to go vegan, but back in the 1880s there were some people who were thought to be very unlikely to ever free their slaves. And did that stop people from accepting that black people are every bit as human as white people are? No way! Through welfarist compromises—like bigger cages, for example—welfarists still acknowledge that animals are our property and that it's okay to exploit them as long as we spare them unnecessary suffering. But when is *any* suffering necessary? When is animal exploitation in any fashion the only option? When one fights for small, incremental changes like promoting cage-free eggs (rather than spend that energy against consumption of eggs, period), one sends the message that exploitation of animals is, at its basis, ethical and acceptable. There's simply no getting around that, and no claiming that that's in line with the true ideals of vegan. People go vegan because they're against animal exploitation in any form and know that the first and biggest step is ending animal exploitation in their own lives. So why, then, do welfarist vegans stay vegan? I mean, if cage-free eggs and free-range meat are such great, humane products that will have such an impact on the end of animal exploitation, why don't welfarists eat them? If they've ended animal exploitation in their own lives, why do they not encourage others to do the same? Welfarism is, in a way, hypocritical. Welfarists say that cage-free eggs and so forth are such great products, such wonderful victories for animals, so ethically acceptable, yet they don't consume cage-free eggs themselves. Our ethics must match our actions and our efforts we put forth must match the ends we desire if our movement is going to get anywhere and mean anything.

Think about history. Were there a bunch of abolitionists sitting around toward the end of the nineteenth century saying, "Well, we can't end slavery now, but in the meantime maybe we can make the boat ride over a little more comfortable"? No way! Can you picture a group of suffragists having a meeting to talk about how they can't get the right to vote anytime soon, but can at least make a few jobs more open to women? No! Nowadays, are there groups that advocate humane rape or human-welfare slavery? Not that I can see. Welfarism admits defeat before even putting up a fight.

Don't get me wrong. I know that it's going to take many small steps over a long period of time to truly liberate animals. But these steps are reducing animal usage in our day-to-day lives and people going vegan, not using warehouses instead of cages. Abolitionists, myself included, are perfectly aware that the battle for animal liberation is going to be a long one in need of a great many people putting forth a great deal of effort. Eradicating slavery in the United States was a huge task, but a small group of dedicated individuals did it. The fight for women's rights was no doubt difficult, but the progress made in the past few centuries has been overwhelming.

Welfarists often accuse abolitionists of not caring about the animals that are suffering now, right this second. If we truly cared about ending animal suffering, they say, why oh why would we *not* want to fight for making an animal's life just the tiniest bit less painful? They assume that we're too wrapped up with ending the whole thing to notice that we can impact how much animals are suffering now. All animal activists, abolitionists included, know that gestation crates suck and that chickens in cages suffer immensely. But while welfarists would rather have animals out of crates and cages but still (truly) suffering, being slaughtered, and being consumed as objects, abolitionists prefer that we fight for animals to not even be born into the hell that humans have created for them.

Animals aren't objects and they're not ours. We can and will end their exploitation. Our efforts have to look like they're efforts towards what we actually say we want, not just the lesser of two evils.

Falling Off the Wagon

So you woke up one morning and your mom was making scrambled eggs. They just looked so good, and there wasn't much else to eat. You figured one little plateful wouldn't be that bad...and now you've got a stomachache and feel like a bad person. You remembered where those eggs came from and feel bad, plus now you're worried about screwing up again. You fell off the vegan wagon.

Well, calm down. I'm not saying that it's okay to eat animals every now and again, but you know, tomorrow is a new day. You *can* have control over your choices and you *can* be vegan. Even if you feel bad about your slip-up, don't dwell on it much. Instead, spend on your energy on thinking about how you're going to stay vegan now. What's done is done and you can either sit around feeling sad or you can learn from it and never have to be sad in that way again. And if you think you're the first person to have a stumble or two before really staying vegan, think again. Once you become accustomed to being vegan, once you know which things to eat and which not to, once you know how to make sure that you don't do something you'll feel bad about later, it's smooth sailing.

If you're really scared you're going to mess up again, there are some things you can do to prevent this. Keep a Luna bar (or some similar food that won't go bad) in your car or backpack at all times. That way, you'll always have something vegan to eat and won't cave to your hunger and pick something not vegan. Emergency snacks like that can be lifesavers! Also, before something tempts you, remind yourself why you want to be vegan. Think about if it's going to be worth it when you're full but feel like a hypocrite. Breathe. Relax. Focus on being vegan for this day, not overwhelming yourself with thoughts of decades and decades of veganism. One day becomes another day becomes another day. Being vegan takes getting used to, but you can do it!

Practical vs. Symbolic Veganism

Veganism is not about purity or following a doctrine or not breaking rules. Veganism is about doing as much as is possible and practical to not support speciesism. No matter how much you want to, it really is impossible to a live a life that is *completely* free of animal products. There are animal products in tires, for example. You'd be hard-pressed to find medicine that is truly vegan.

Even fruits, vegetables, and grains (as defensive omnis love to point out) will probably kill a few mice as they're being harvested. But does this mean you have to stop driving or taking medicine, or that you shouldn't eat fruit? Not at all. Does it mean that since you can't be 100 percent animal-free in your life, you should give up and eat animal products sometimes? Not at all.

Do what's possible and do what's practical. It's more than possible to avoid crackers with whey in them. It's definitely practical to use soymilk in your coffee. You don't need crackers or creamy coffee to live. It's not possible or practical to avoid medication that contains animal products or is tested on animals. If you need medicine to live, take it! The vegan police, I promise you, are not going to show up on your doorstep to scream at you about what a bad person you are to choose to save your life/health instead of suffering. It's also not really practical to avoid some very, very small traces of animal products. I don't mean whey or beeswax. I mean, if you refuse to eat products that don't have the Certified Vegan label on them and are not made by vegans for vegans on 100 percent vegan equipment, more power to ya, but that does more harm (to you) than good (to the world). If you eat like that, you're not going to be eating much. Plus, you make it seem like veganism is all about deprival. Certain "vegan" groups use that argument to justify eating small amounts of animal products, like whey, but that's not deprival, that's, um, *veganism*.

The vast majority of vegans agree on issues like medicine, but with certain products, it gets gray. For example, some sugar is refined using char from animal bones. So some vegans don't eat refined sugar because there is a possibility that it might have been made *with* animal products, even if the animal products are not actually present in the sugar. Some vegans, like me, see this more as a symbolic act not particularly worth much energy. If I know for a fact that this kind of sugar is refined using bone char, I won't eat it, but I'm not going to kill myself trying to find out how every grain of sugar I eat is refined. I just think my thoughts and effort are going to be used better in other ways. I'm the same way with other really very tiny "animal products." Glycerin that I don't know the source of? Won't eat it. Some random vitamin that I don't know the source of? Will. It's completely possible to avoid bigger things like glycerin. Some smaller things like that just aren't possible to avoid all the time, and that's just how it is. Am I still vegan? Yeah. Does this justify eating other animal products? No, because that's not vegan, because it's possible and practical to avoid the vast majority of animal-derived ingredients.

Part Three:
Food

CHAPTER NINE: WHAT VEGANS REALLY EAT

★

If I had a penny for every non-vegan who has ever wondered what the hell vegans really eat, or thought it was only tofu and salad, I could definitely buy a lifetime supply of vegan ice cream sandwiches for me and all the other vegans in the world. If you're a new vegan, you've probably contributed to that fund, and that's okay, but now you're not just wondering for the sake of wondering, you're wondering because you're hungry. Worry not, because if you're thinking that you're going to be eating salad for breakfast, nothing for lunch, and scraped-off side dishes for dinner, it's time to change your mind.

Breakfast shouldn't be that hard. There are delicious and nutritious vegan alternatives to non-vegan breakfast foods you may be used to. Many cereals (even a lot of the sugary, popular ones) are "accidentally vegan" and you can just pour soy, rice, almond milk, or one of the other many vegan milks out there on top of it. Scour your local healthfood store for brands of vegan waffles, because they do exist, or find a recipe and make your own. Same for pancakes—a surprising amount of regular mixes are vegan and you can simply use nondairy milk/butter with them. Make toast and spread it with jelly, peanut butter, or vegan butter/margarine. Make a smoothie with fruit and soy yogurt. Spread a bagel with vegan cream cheese or peanut butter. Have a bowl of oatmeal (most brands are vegan) with dried fruit and peanut or cashew butter in it. Being vegan means you're automatically a hippie, obviously, so prove it and try some granola. Scramble tofu with spices and veggies (see page 124 for my recipe). Take that scrambled tofu and throw it in a tortilla with potatoes and vegan sausage for a breakfast burrito. Top a rice cake with nut butter and fruit. Fruit by itself is always a good, light, healthy breakfast. Make muffins the night before and heat a few up in the morning. Break out of the breakfast mold and just heat up leftovers from the night before—I love having miso soup for breakfast. If you're in a hurry, take a banana and a bag of dry vegan cereal with you—take a bite of the banana and then dip it in the cereal, it'll stick. You can also find individual juicebox-style soymilk cartons to take with you. See, that was easy! One meal down!

Lunch may not seem as easy as breakfast because now you're at school. A full morning of classes and you're ready to march into the lunchroom, whip out your wallet, and have some nice...uh, deep-fried flesh sandwich? Not vegan. Nachos drowning in fluorescent cow pus? Not vegan. Peanut butter and jelly? Hmm. Suspicious bread. No. Iceberg lettuce? Vegan, but boring and gross and void of any nutrition whatsoever.

The cafeteria is a dangerous place. At some high schools (like my former) the vegan pickings are incredibly slim. I could get pretzels, plain chips, or *one* of the many fruit plates, with the possibility of a PB&J, depending on the bread. *Score.* I assume and, for the sake of humankind, hope that some high schools are more vegan-friendly, but somehow I think that might not be the case.

The school lunch program started off to provide use for the USDA's surplus foods, in a time when meat, dairy, and eggs were considered among the healthiest of foods. Today's school lunches follow loose nutritional guidelines and base their meals primarily around meat and dairy products, with most grains being refined and white, and few fruits/vegetables. While most middle and high school cafeterias have many options other than the school lunch, it tends to be junk food.

So what's a vegan teen to do? You can:
   A. Live off potato chips and ~~crunchy water~~
      iceberg lettuce
   B. Pack your lunch!

If you want to choose A, be aware that you're most likely going to become The Unhealthy Vegan (you know, with arms close to the color and thickness of pencils) and give the impression that veganism means deprival and not much else.

If you want to choose B, be aware that you'll be as healthy as you want to be, can pack things so good you'll look forward to them all morning, and still have extra time in the morning if you need it. Keep reading!

Brown-bagging it is the way to go. Well, really, it's not, because brown bags are not so great. You have to keep buying them, they're wasteful, they look boring, and they won't keep things cold if you want them to. I recommend investing in a really good reusable lunchbox/bag, and some reusable plastic food containers in different sizes are great, too. Get a lunchbox that's nice and sturdy, with at least some insulation. My lunchbag is nicely insulated, easy to clean, and even says "No Animals In Here" on it. That's the only AR-message lunchbag I've seen, but if you poke around at toy stores and garage sales I'm sure you can find something with robots or dinosaurs or something if you're scenexcore like that.

Taking your lunch, however, is great. You get to control what you eat, you don't have to wait in any lines, and it's cheaper than buying your lunch every day. Plus, when you're vegan, taking your lunch means the difference between an empty, sad belly and a full, happy one. If you're usually short on time in the mornings, pack your lunch the night before and stick it in the fridge, then in the morning you can simply grab it. Below is a guide to start making a perfect vegan packed lunch. Use the tables to craft any number of basic lunchy things, vegan-style.

Sandwiches, Wraps, etc.

Starchy Things:

* Tortilla
* Sliced bread
* Crusty roll
* Flavored wrap
* Pita pocket
* Bagel

Spreads:

* Vegan mayo
* Hummus
* Baba ghanouj
* Peanut, cashew, or almond butter
* Tahini
* Vegan marshmallow fluff

* Jelly or jam
* Agave or rice nectar

Veggies/Fruits:

* Spinach
* Pepper slices
* Mushrooms
* Matchstick carrots
* Dried cranberries
* Apple slices

High-protein:

* Vegan cold cuts
* Tofu, seitan, or tempeh
* Pine nuts, cashews, or other nuts

Salads

Base:

* Spinach
* Lettuce
* Bok choy
* Kale
* Romaine
* Arugula or red leaf lettuce

Dressing:

* Vegan Honey Mustard (page 123)
* Vegan ranch
* Italian

* Balsamic vinaigrette

Random:

* Pine nuts, cashews, or other nuts
* Tofu, seitan, tempeh
* Matchstick carrots
* Mushrooms, peppers, or other veggies
* Dried cranberries
* Mandarin oranges
* Chow mein noodles
* Nutritional yeast
* Crumbles of vegan cheese

Last night's leftovers are also a typical lunch for me. In fact, thinking about this past school year, I took two or three salads total, a sandwich maybe once every two weeks, and the rest of the time leftovers from dinner. Having good reusable food containers helps in the lunch-taking process immensely. But what do vegans eat for dinner?

More than salad, that's for sure. Not that salad isn't great and healthy. But salad is just one of the many, many things that vegans eat for dinner. A vegan cookbook, or even a veganized recipe from a non-vegan cookbook, is a great place to start. Turn to page 75 for a list. But you don't necessarily need a cookbook every night. Like with breakfast, in most cases you can simply replace what you used to eat with its vegan equivalent, and there are also a lot of delicious vegan dishes that don't rely on these substitutes. Use mock beef crumbles in pasta sauce instead of beef, or just leave them out. Make quesadillas or burritos with roasted vegetables and beans. Have a bowl of soup made with veggie broth instead of chicken or beef broth. Top a baked potato with vegan sour cream, vegan butter, broccoli, mock bacon bits, nutritional yeast, or whatever other toppings you can think of. Stir-fry veggies with rice or noodles and teriyaki sauce. Make veggie and seitan kabobs. Use beans in chili instead of meat. Explore different ethnic foods you may not have tried, like Indian, Mediterranean, Thai, or Japanese food. Peanut butter and jelly is a classic. Mashed potatoes can be made with vegan butter and nondairy milk. Replace chicken with seitan in casseroles. Use silken tofu instead of eggs in quiche recipes. If you want comfort food, try macaroni and vegan cheese. Roast potatoes with olive oil, rosemary, pepper, and salt. Marinate tempeh in barbeque sauce. Have a sandwich with vegan lunchmeat slices. Grill portobello mushrooms and serve between buns with fries.

Snacks are important too. For some yummy, quick vegan snacks that are even on the healthy side (mostly), try: popcorn with nutritional yeast (Act II brand Butter

Lover's is ironically vegan, or make your own), grapes, bananas, pretzels, granola/energy bars, fruit leathers, melon, a bagel half with peanut butter, soy yogurt, frozen juice bars, trail mix, peaches, applesauce, crackers, oranges, pita/veggies and hummus, cherries, chips and salsa, peanuts, cashews, almonds, or other nuts, dried fruit, oven fries, apples and peanut butter, sandwiches, cereal, rice cakes, plums, muffins, vegan ice cream sandwiches, graham crackers, vegan nachos, salad, or rice crisps.

CHAPTER TEN: NEW FOODS

★

One day I was sitting in French class, when my teacher started asking me about what I ate and did not eat. I told her that I didn't eat meat, dairy, or eggs, and she was so shocked that she went back to speaking to me in English. "You do not eat any of it?" she asked. I shook my head. "Well, like, what *do* you eat?" "Everything but that!" I told her. "Yeah, but that's not much!"

My teacher thinks like most non-vegan people do. The idea of cutting out three major categories of food seems like it would make your diet incredibly limited, a never-ending rotation of dry salad and limp veggie burgers. However, I've found the exact opposite to be true—because I no longer ate animal products, I had to find things to eat instead, and the variety of my diet grew incredibly. It seems funny to me now that omnivores who supposedly eat "everything" limit their diets so much by only sticking to foods familiar to them. As I explored new vegan foods, things I had never eaten, seen, or heard of became favorites of mine. Maybe your pregan diet was more varied than mine, but I'm sure there are at least a few things on this list that you haven't tried yet.

Nutritional Yeast is an inactive form of yeast—don't confuse it with brewer's yeast—that has a cheesy, somewhat nutty flavor. It's yellow and you can buy it in bulk at health food stores in large or small flakes. Nutritional yeast is also a great source of vitamin B12 if you get the fortified kind (like Red Star Vegetarian Supplement). It can be used in a ton of different ways, but I like to sprinkle it on popcorn, make a cheezy sauce out of it (see page 121), top pasta or veggies with it, put it on toast or bagels...basically, anything that can hold the stuff is a good use for it. Get creative. I've even had a peanut butter and nutritional yeast sandwich, but I'm weird.

Tofu is an incredibly versatile soy product that comes in blocks. It is pretty bland by itself, but it's not meant to be eaten that way. Tofu absorbs the flavor of whatever you marinate it in or cook it with. Use firm and extra-firm varieties in stir-fries, grilling, baking, or wherever you would use meat. Use silken in smoothies, dips, puddings, and other desserts. Tofu is a good source of manganese, iron, protein, calcium (if it's calcium-set), and many other nutrients. You can find tofu at virtually any grocery store, whether it's the health-food kind or not.

Tempeh (TEM-pay) is another soy product you can use in place of meat. Tempeh is made of both soy and mushrooms and has a meatier texture than tofu. Tempeh is a good substitute for chicken and also makes great vegan bacon. It's a good source of manganese, copper, protein, vitamin B2, and other nutrients.

Seitan, (SAY-tan) or "wheat meat" is a meat (usually poultry) substitute made with the protein from wheat. Making your own is tastier, but you can find it in most health food stores. Seitan is the basis for most prepackaged fake meats. Use it anywhere you would use chicken.

Hummus is a Middle Eastern spread/dip made of chickpeas and tahini (sesame seed paste). You can find it in most regular grocery stores, and it comes in lots of flavors—I've seen everything from roasted red pepper to avocado to curry. Hummus and pita bread go the best together, but dipping chips and pretzels into it is great, too. It's also a good spread for a wrap (see page 121). Hummus is a good source of fiber, healthy fat, protein, iron, and yumminess!

TVP may not sound like food, but it is. TVP stands for Textured Vegetable Protein. Basically, it's the protein in vegetables that has been isolated, dehydrated, put into chunks, and sold to you. It absorbs the liquid you cook it in to be like little chunks of nonflavored meat, but like tofu it takes on the flavor of whatever you cook it with. Especially great for making sloppy joes (page 126)!

Falafel is another dish from the Mediterranean. Falafel are patties or balls made of spiced chickpeas. They are usually eaten in a pita with lettuce, tomato, and tahini.

Fruits/Vegetables you may not have tried: golden kiwis, pluots, persimmons, lychees, pomegranates, pomelos, kumquats, mangos, kale, jicama, or chard!

Couscous is Middle Eastern and is basically pasta dough rolled into very tiny spheres. You can buy plain couscous in bulk or flavored and faster-cooking couscous in boxes. Couscous is traditionally served under a meat or vegetable stew.

Samosas are Indian and consist of a pastry shell filled with potatoes, peas, onions, curry spices and sometimes meat. Frozen samosas—even ones with tofu—are becoming common in the U.S.

Curry is a spicy, sauce-based dish from South Asia (but mainly India). Most, but not all, curries are made with either curry leaves or curry powder. Curries are usually eaten with rice and meat or vegetables.

Quinoa (KEEN-wah) is a South American grain. It is one of the few plant foods that contain all nine essential amino acids. If you aren't using boxed quinoa, rinse it first. Once cooked, quinoa has a mild, nutty flavor and is a good alternative to rice, couscous, or other grains.

Amaranth is a Latin American grain. You can toast it and it's just like very, very small popcorn. Amaranth also contains all nine essential amino acids, not that that really matters.

Tahini is a paste of ground sesame seeds, with a consistency similar to peanut butter. Tahini is used in making hummus and is also common in Middle Eastern sauces.

Soymilk is a milky drink made from soybeans and water. It has nutritional value similar to cow's milk and is just one of many vegan alternatives (others include rice, almond, hemp, oat, and nut) to moo juice. Soymilk can be found in all groceries and most coffee shops. It comes in a variety of flavors—from vanilla and strawberry to chai and eggnog! Fun fact: when you curdle and ferment soymilk, you get tofu!

Miso is a Japanese paste made from the fermentation of salt with rice, barley, and/or soybeans. It's usually salty and it is most commonly used (at least outside of Japan) to make miso soup, a salty soup usually featuring tofu, noodles, and seaweed. Watch out, though—miso soup can be found vegan, but it usually is made from fish stock!

CHAPTER ELEVEN: THE RECIPES

Easy, yummy, by a vegan teen for vegan teens. Most of these I don't measure out, so use your own judgment when it calls for a "glop" or a "good shake" of something. These recipes aren't concrete—feel free to change them however you want.

Hummus

Sure, the already-prepared stuff you buy in the grocery is great, but you should try making it for yourself at least once, or else you won't get your vegan ID card. *So* good. If you don't have tahini, peanut or other nut butters can work, and it's pretty hard to give this a bad combination of spices.

* 1 (15.5 oz.) can chickpeas
* Juice of 1 lemon
* 1 tablespoon minced garlic
* 1 tablespoon olive oil
* Good shake of pepper
* 1 tablespoon water
* 1 tablespoon tahini

Combine all ingredients in a food processor until smooth. Serve with pita bread and veggies.

Cheezy Sauce

This recipe was adapted from a mac 'n' cheeze recipe in *La Dolce Vegan!*

* 3 tablespoons vegan butter/margarine
* 3 tablespoons flour
* Salt and pepper
* 1½ cups ricemilk or other milk
* ¼ to ½ cup nutritional yeast

In a small saucepan, melt the butter. Remove from heat, add the flour, and mix until it becomes a thick paste. Return to medium heat and add ½ cup of the ricemilk, whisking constantly, until it becomes thick and smooth. Repeat two more times with the remaining ricemilk, then add the nutritional yeast, salt, and pepper. Whisk again, and serve over pasta or veggies.

Peanut Sauce

This is one of my vegan staples. When I'm feeling lazy and uncreative, I make this with rice and veggies or vegan chicken, though it's good on pretty much anything.

* Glop of peanut butter
* 1 tablespoon teriyaki sauce
* Garlic powder to taste
* Water

Melt the peanut butter in a small saucepan over medium-low heat. Remove from heat and add teriyaki and garlic powder. Stir. Slowly add water, stirring constantly, until it's a lighter consistency than peanut butter and has a gravy-like consistency. Serves 1 or 2.

Hummus Addict Salad Dressing

There's a little hummus addict in all of us, and this recipe is much healthier than pretty much any other salad dressing out there.

* A few tablespoons hummus
* A few tablespoons water
* Salt, black pepper, and garlic to taste (optional)

Combine the hummus and water in a small dish and stir until smooth, creamy, and drizzle-able. Add the other seasonings and stir. Pour over salad and eat. Serves 1.

Vegan Honey Mustard Dressing

The best friend of spinach and vegan chicken.

* One part Dijon mustard (make sure it's vegan)
* One part agave nectar or rice nectar

Stir both ingredients until thoroughly combined.

Tomato-Alfredo Sauce

This was inspired by two recipes from the blog Vegan Yum Yum. This is good for a special occasion or just when you're feeling special yourself.

* 1 cup soymilk
* 1/3 cup raw, unsalted cashews
* 1/4 cup nutritional yeast
* 3 tablespoons soy sauce or Bragg's
* 2 tablespoons vegan butter
* 1 tablespoon tahini
* 1 tablespoon lemon juice
* 2 teaspoon Dijon mustard
* 1/2 teaspoon paprika
* Pinch nutmeg
* 2 to 4 cloves garlic (optional)
* Freshly ground black pepper
* 3 tablespoons tomato paste
* Small handful grape tomatoes or half a regular tomato
* 1/2 tablespoon basil

Combine all ingredients in a food processor or blender until smooth. Because of the raw cashews, it probably won't be completely smooth, but do your best and don't worry about it if there are a few cashew bits. Pour into a saucepan and cook on medium heat, stirring, until warm and thickened. Serve over pasta. Serves 2 to 3.

Ultimate Nachos

Even more ultimate because they're vegan. This is a messy fiesta.

* Cheezy Sauce (page 121)
* 1 tablespoon chili powder
* 1/2 (I5.5 oz) can black beans
* 3 tablespoons vegan sour
* cream
* 1/2 cup finely shredded lettuce
* Tortilla chips

Combine cheezy sauce with chili powder and pour over tortilla chips. Top with remaining ingredients. Serves 1.

Snack Mix

Combine any of the following for an easy and relatively healthy after-school snack.

* Sesame sticks
* Dried cranberries
* Dried coconut flakes
* Cereal

* Walnuts, peanuts, cashews, almonds, etc.
* Vegan chocolate chips

Tofu Scrambler

Every vegan should know how to make a good tofu scrambler. Feel free to play with this recipe as much as you like.

* 2 teaspoon oil
* Half a medium onion, chopped
* 2 teaspoon turmeric
* 1 teaspoon garlic powder
* 2 teaspoon soy sauce, tamari, or Bragg's
* 2 teaspoon freshly ground black pepper

* 2 teaspoon paprika
* 2 teaspoon basil
* ¼ cup nutritional yeast
* 1 (16-oz.) block firm tofu, crumbled
* 1 cup hash browns
* 2 or 3 baby carrots, finely chopped

Heat the oil in a skillet. Add onion and sauté for 2 to 3 minutes, until soft. Add all the seasonings, then add the tofu. Stir it around to get everything mixed up, then cook on medium heat for about 5 minutes. Add the hash browns, stir, and cook for another 10 to 12 minutes. Add the carrots and cook for another minute. Serves 2.

Chili

If you think chili simply must have meat, prepare to find out how wrong you are...in a most delicious fashion.

* 2 (15.5 oz.) cans beans, two different kinds (I like black and chili), drained and rinsed
* 1 can vegetable broth
* 1 bell pepper, diced
* Cumin powder to taste

* Garlic powder to taste
* Onion powder to taste
* Freshly ground black pepper to taste
* TVP, amount varies depending on how "meaty" you want it

Combine all ingredients in a large saucepan. Bring to a boil and cook for at least 10 minutes, until the TVP is thoroughly cooked. Serves 4.

White Bean Stew

This is the first recipe that my mom veganized so she would have something to cook for me. How sweet. This is delicious on a cold night!

* 1 tablespoon olive oil
* 1 medium onion, chopped
* 1 jalapeño pepper, seeded and chopped
* 4 cloves garlic, minced
* 2 cans veggie broth
* 1¼ teaspoons cumin
* 2 (15.5 oz) cans cannellini beans
* 2 tablespoons flour
* ¼ cup cold water
* 2 tablespoons chopped fresh cilantro

In a large soup pot, heat the oil. Sauté the onion, jalapeño, and garlic until tender. Add the broth, beans, and cumin. Bring to a boil, then reduce heat and cover. Simmer for 10 to 15 minutes. Combine flour and water until smooth, stir into stew. Bring to a boil again, and cook while stirring for 2 minutes, until thickened. Add cilantro, heat through, and serve. Serves 6.

Veghettios

I'm still holding out for the canned vegan version of the childhood favorite, but in the meantime this is a pretty good substitute taste-wise. You can also put this in the food processor and make a good pasta sauce that has the added nutritional punch of chickpeas.

* 1 can chickpeas, undrained
* ⅔ cup tomato/marinara sauce
* 1 teaspoon minced garlic
* Black pepper
* At least ½ teaspoon oregano
* 1 tablespoon nutritional yeast

Don't drain the chickpeas, and pour them into a saucepan. Take out a few tablespoons of the liquid. Add all the other ingredients and stir well. Heat on medium-high until the sauce begins to boil, about 2 to 4 minutes. Serves 2.

Roasted Chickpeas

If you have never roasted a chickpea before, you may as well have never seen the sun rise. Seriously. They become crispy on the outside and tender on the inside, and are addictive.

* 1 can chickpeas, drained and rinsed
* 2 tablespoons oil, or enough to coat
* Salt, pepper, garlic, and other seasonings to taste

Preheat oven to 450º F. Combine all ingredients in a bowl and stir until evenly mixed. Pour into a baking pan with a lip (very important). Bake for about 20 to 25 minutes until golden brown and crispy. Serves 2.

Random Vegetable Joy

Fresh. Healthy. Goes well with noodles/rice and peanut sauce.

* Handful of frozen edamame
* Handful of cremini mushrooms, sliced or chopped
* Handful of broccoli florets
* One small can of pineapple tidbits
* At least one of the following:
* 1 teaspoon sesame oil
* 1 tablespoon soy sauce

Put the edamame in a bowl of water and microwave for at least a minute. Combine with the remaining ingredients in a small skillet and sauté for at least 5 to 10 minutes. Serves 2.

Sloppy Joes

My dad goes crazy for these and insists that I make them every time I am home. They are *good*. The amounts below are estimates—you must follow your own inner sloppy joe artist to get the best combination.

* 1 cup TVP
* 1½ cups water
* 2 tablespoons liquid smoke
* 1 tablespoon garlic powder
* 1 tablespoon onion powder
* 1 tablespoon apple juice (optional but so good)
* 3 tablespoons ketchup
* ½ cup barbeque sauce

Combine the TVP and water in a medium-sized pan. Add the remaining ingredients and mix thoroughly. Cook until the TVP has absorbed almost all of the liquid and is tender and reddish-brown. Mmmmm. Serves 6.

Veggie Fried Rice

This is great for weekend mornings that start at about one in the afternoon—it's really pretty easy to throw together but you feel like a productive, actual-meal-cooking member of society, and you get more vegetables in your belly from brunch, or whatever it is you're eating, than a lot of omnivores get in a whole day.

* 1 cup rice
* 1 red bell pepper
* 1 cup broccoli florets
* Six or more mushrooms, preferably cremini
* About six baby carrots
* 1 teaspoon sesame oil
* Small handful of cashews
* 2 tablespoons soy or teriyaki sauce, divided
* 1 teaspoon garlic powder
* 1 teaspoon onion powder

Cook the rice according to directions on package/rice maker. As rice is cooking, dice the pepper, cut the carrots into coins, and slice the mushrooms. Add the oil to a large skillet and cook the carrots for 2 minutes. Add the pepper and cook for 2 minutes more. Add the mushrooms and cook for 2 minutes more. Add cashews and 1 tablespoon soy sauce. Add the rice and the rest of the soy sauce. Serves 2 to 4.

The Easiest Brownies

These brownies are the best thing in the world. For one, you make them in the microwave. Hello, college. For another, if you use water instead of soymilk, they are made only with ingredients that any home, vegan or non-, would have.

* 1 banana, mashed
* ¼ cup vegetable oil
* 1 teaspoon vanilla
* 3 tablespoons water or chocolate soymilk
* ¾ cup sugar
* 1 cup flour
* 4 tablespoons cocoa
* ½ teaspoon salt
* chocolate chips

Combine the banana, oil, vanilla, and water/soymilk. Add the sugar, flour, cocoa, salt, and chocolate chips. Mix until there are no large lumps, then pour into a greased, microwave-safe dish. Microwave on high for 4 to 6 minutes, then let sit, covered but out of the microwave, for another 10 minutes or so.

No-Knead Bread

This recipe is a little time-intensive, but most of it is time when you're waiting for it to rise and can be doing something else. You don't need to knead this bread, which makes it ridiculously easy, but it's still as fluffy as bread you do knead and makes your house smell just as amazing.

* ¼ cup warm water
* 2 (0.25 oz.) packets yeast
* 2 cups hot water
* 3 tablespoons sugar
* 1 tablespoon salt
* 6 cups flour
* ⅓ cup vegetable oil

Pour the warm water into a small bowl and add the yeast, but don't stir. Set aside.

In a large mixing bowl, pour the hot water over the sugar and salt, then stir to completely dissolve. Combine 3 cups of the flour with the water mixture. Pour the oil on top of the dough mixture, then add the yeast mixture on top of that, but don't stir. Top with the remaining 3 cups of the flour and mix well, using your hands if you need to. At this point, the dough should be pliant and moist, but not gooey. Cover the bowl with a damp towel and set aside somewhere warm to rise for at least 45 minutes. On a lightly floured cutting board or countertop, divide the dough into half. flatten each half into roughly an oval/rounded rectangular shape, about ½- to ¾-inch thickness; then roll the dough lengthwise and place on an ungreased cookie sheet. Cover the dough with a moist towel and set aside somewhere warm to rise for another 45 minutes. After the dough has risen the second time, preheat the oven to 375º F and bake for 20 minutes. Let cool and enjoy! Makes two big loaves.

Pudding

Creamy, chocolatey, full of calcium, B12, and joy. This is a favorite of mine for a late-night snack.

* ½ cup chocolate soymilk
* 1 tablespoons cornstarch
* 1 tablespoon sweetened cocoa powder

Combine all ingredients in a small saucepan.

Cook on medium heat until thickened, whisking constantly.

When thick, turn off the heat and continue whisking until cooled (otherwise it will be lumpy). Serves 1.

Chocolate Banana Milkshake

This is so healthy, so delicious, and so easy. During the summer I usually have one of these a day. Yum.

* 1 banana, sliced and frozen
* 1 cup of chocolate soymilk
* 1 tablespoon peanut butter (optional)
* 1 teaspoon cinnamon (optional)

Combine all ingredients in blender and blend until smooth. Serves one.

Some Vegan Kitchen Wisdom

Egg replacers allow you to veganize standard recipes for baked goods. Different recipes use eggs for different things, so one kind of egg replacer may work wonderfully in this recipe but not so great in another. Experiment. For one egg, you can use any of the following:

* 1 teaspoon egg replacer powder (buy this at health food stores, one box will last you your entire life) plus 2 tablespoons warm water
* ½ mashed banana, 1 tablespoon ground flaxseeds plus 2 tablespoons water
* 1 tablespoon soy flour plus 2 tablespoons water
* ¼ cup soy yogurt or ¼ cup applesauce plus 1 teaspoon baking powder

Oven temperatures actually vary from oven to oven, and this can have a big impact on whatever you're baking. If time after time your baked goods come out burnt or undercooked, consider buying a stand-alone oven thermometer to find out the difference between what you're setting your oven to and what the oven's temperature actually is.

When you're cooking, **clean as you go**. If something needs to cook by itself for a few minutes, put away the dishes and ingredients you no longer need, or put one thing away as you get another thing out. **Multitask**, too. If you're making pasta, for example, make the sauce or chop the veggies while the water boils.

Things worth the time and effort: grilling your pita bread (brush with olive oil first), making your own tortilla chips (cut a tortilla into bite-sized pieces, spray with cooking spray and bake at 375º for ten minutes or so), getting quality ingredients for a special recipe, having a good knife, using in-season produce, and trying new things.

Part Four:
Now Stay Vegan!

Chapter Twelve: Inspire Me, Please

Great Quotes

"Be who you are and say what you feel, because those who mind don't matter and those who matter don't mind."
—*Dr. Seuss*

"There are a thousand hacking at the branches of evil to one who is striking at the roots."
—*Henry David Thoreau*

"Our lives begin to end the day we become silent about things that matter."
—*Martin Luther King*

"You must be the change you wish to see in the world."
—*Mahatma Gandhi*

"I have no doubt that it is a part of the destiny of the human race, in its gradual improvement, to leave off eating animals"
—*Henry David Thoreau*

"It is my view that the vegetarian manner of living by its purely physical effect on the human temperament would most beneficially influence the lot of mankind."
—*Albert Einstein*

"Do not let what you cannot do interfere with what you can do."
—*John Wooden*

"The greatness of a nation and its moral progress can be judged by the way its animals are treated."
—*Mahatma Gandhi*

"How good it is to be well-fed, healthy, and kind all at the same time."
—*Henry J. Heimlich*

"Anger is an energy!"
—*John Lydon*

"A man can live and be healthy without killing animals for food; therefore, if he eats meat, he participates in taking of animal life merely for the sake of his appetite. And to act so is immoral."

—*Leo Tolstoy*

"Power to act is duty to act."

—*Peter Kropotkin*

"The world, we are told, was made especially for man—a presumption not supported by all the facts... Why should man value himself as more than a small part of the one great unit of creation?"

—*John Muir*

"All truth passes through three stages. First, it is ridiculed. Second, it is violently opposed. Third, it is accepted as self-evident."

—*Arthur Schopenhauer*

"Wild animals never kill for sport. Man is the only one to whom the torture and death of his fellow creatures is amusing in itself."

—*James A. Froud*

"If one person is unkind to an animal it is considered to be cruelty, but where a lot of people are unkind to animals, especially in the name of commerce, the cruelty is condoned and, once large sums of money are at stake, will be defended to the last by otherwise intelligent people."

—*Ruth Harrison*

"What is it that should trace the insuperable line? The question is not, Can they reason? nor Can they talk? but, Can they suffer?"

—*Jeremy Bentham*

"Each snowflake in an avalanche pleads not guilty."

—*Stanislaw J. Lec*

"The worst sin toward our fellow creatures is not to hate them, but to be indifferent to them: that's the essence of inhumanity."

—*George Bernard Shaw*

"Cowardice asks the question, 'Is it safe?' Expediency asks the question, 'Is it politic?' Vanity asks the question, 'Is it popular?' But conscience asks the question, 'Is it right?' And there comes a time when one must take a position that is neither safe, nor politic, nor popular; but one must take it because it is right."

—*Martin Luther King*

"Unless someone like you cares a whole awful lot, nothing is going to get better, it's not."

—*Dr. Seuss*

"Truly man is the king of beasts, for his brutality exceeds them. We live by the death of others. We are burial places. I have from an early age abjured the use of meat, and the time will come when men such as I will look on the murder of animals as they now look on the murder of men."

—*Leonardo da Vinci*

"The animals of the world exist for their own reasons. They were not made for humans any more than black people were made for white, or women created for men."

—*Alice Walker*

"As long as men massacre animals, they will kill each other. Indeed, he who sows the seeds of murder and pain cannot reap the joy of love."

—*Pythagoras*

"I don't understand why asking people to eat a well-balanced vegetarian diet is considered drastic, while it is medically conservative to cut people open."

—*Dean Ornish, M.D.*

"As long as there is conscious life on Earth, there will be suffering. The question becomes what to do with the existence each of us is given. We can choose to add our own fury and misery to the rest, or we can set an example by simultaneously working constructively to alleviate suffering while leading joyous, meaningful, fulfilled lives. Being a vegan isn't about deprivation or anger. It's about being fully aware so as to be fully alive."

—*Matt Ball, Vegan Outreach*

"When a human being kills an animal for food, he is neglecting his own hunger for justice. Man prays for mercy, but is unwilling to extend it to others. Why then should man expect mercy from God? It is unfair to expect something that you are not willing to give."

—*Isaac Bashevis Singer*

"In matters of conscience, the law of majority has no place."

—*Mahatma Gandhi*

"The conventional view serves to protect us from the painful job of thinking."

—*John Kenneth Galbraith*

"It's a matter of taking the side of the weak against the strong, something the best people have always done."

—*Harriet Beecher Stowe*

"Sometimes you have to laugh. And sometimes you have to stop laughing and start fighting back."

—*Will Potter*

"Ultimately, an unbiased observer of human behavior must conclude that most action is not shaped by theory, but rather theories are shaped to conform to actions we have no intention of changing."
—Marjorie Spiegel

"Loyalty to a petrified opinion never yet broke a chain or freed a human soul."
—Mark Twain

"Veganism is an ethic that is committed to reverence and respect for all life and the planet that sustains it. Veganism brings with it the joy of living with peace of spirit, and the comfort of knowing that one's thoughts, feelings, words, and actions have a strongly benevolent effect on the world."
—Stanley Sapon

"There is nothing more frightful than ignorance in action."
—Johann Wolfgang von Goethe

"We are the movement and every one of us is so important. Without any one of us the movement is weaker and poorer for the loss. Without all of us the movement ceases to exist. Who will then care about the animals?"
—Barry Horne

"Can you really ask what reason Pythagoras had for abstaining from flesh? For my part I rather wonder both by what accident and in what state of soul or mind the first man did so, touched his mouth to gore and brought his lips to the flesh of a dead creature, he who set forth tables of dead, stale bodies and ventured to call food and nourishment the parts that had a little before bellowed and cried, moved and lived. How could his eyes endure the slaughter when throats were slit and hides flayed and limbs torn from limb? How could his nose endure the stench? How was it that the pollution did not turn away his taste, which made contact with the sores of others and sucked juices and serums from mortal wounds?"
—Plutarch

"The truth will set you free. But first, it will piss you off."
—Gloria Steinem

"Each person must live their life as a model for others."
—Rosa Parks

"I don't pretend to have all the answers, but I react when something's wrong, instead of mindlessly engaging in this corporate sing-along"
—Humanifesto

"Did I do anything wrong today... or has the world always been like this and I've been too wrapped up in myself to notice?"
— *Douglas Adams,*
The Hitchhiker's Guide
to the Galaxy

"And if I don't try, I'm gonna fall into the hatred of this world."
— *The Inside Outs*

"Take sides. Neutrality helps the oppressor, never the victim. Silence encourages the tormentor, never the tormented."
— *Elie Wiesel*

"I am not competing in a popularity contest. On the contrary: it is my function as an ecological activist to say things that people don't want to hear and to do things that people don't want to see done."
— *Captain Paul Watson*

"Never doubt your ability to single handedly change the world. Each of you can move mountains within our political landscape and with your hands mold a brighter future for every living thing. That is not cliché, it's not esoteric, it's real."
— *Andy Stepanian, convicted*
for violating the Animal
Enterprise Terrorism Act by
helping run a news website

"But where was I to start? The world is so vast, I shall start with the country I knew best, my own. But my country is so very large. I had better start with my town. But my town, too, is large. I had best start with my street. No, my home. No, my family. Never mind, I shall start with myself."
— *Elie Wiesel*

Why Vegan Teenagers Kick Ass

Clear skin. All the hormones in meat, dairy, and eggs aggravate your skin. Non-vegan skin cleansers and such are typically harsher than vegan ones. So, going vegan means that you're being easier on your skin from the inside and out. When I went vegan I noticed a big improvement in my skin!

College applications. When you write your essays to get into college, they often want you to write about a personal turning point, something you really care about, a life-changing experience, etc. Cough, cough. Veganism.

Nobody eats your food. Upon first glance, that might seem like a bad thing, but in some cases…it's not! If you live with omnis, even if they like your food, you can get your vegan ice cream straight out of the carton without anybody caring. If you make something extra-fabulous for dinner, the leftovers are going to be there for your lunch.

Maturity. When you're young but old enough on the inside to tackle serious ethical issues—especially when those issues are opposed and ignored by the mainstream—it says something about you. People learn to take you more seriously.

Tendency to question. Questioning one thing (like why we eat animals) leads to questioning other things and, unfortunately, in today's world questioning is a much better habit to get into than blind acceptance. Before I was vegan, I had the mindset that if everyone was doing something, it must be okay, and if everyone believed something, it must be right. Now, I am much better at thinking critically—outside of my time, my upbringing, and what the majority believes—and realizing how I really feel about something.

Inner peace. It's incredibly nice, after you've learned about the horrors of animal exploitation, to have the knowledge that you aren't participating in it at all. Your life is in line with your ethics, you have pulled out of something detestable, you are living a much less violent life. That knowledge can bring great inner peace. No matter how infantile the asshats are being, how little that server knows of what the word *vegan* means, or how disgusting meaty commercials are, vegans can close their eyes and think about the good they are doing for the world and for themselves. And as crunchy as it sounds, I do feel more connected with the world now that I don't eat animals.

More energy! My daily energy levels now are pretty constant now that I've been vegan for a while, but when I first made the switch I noticed a big, positive difference in the amount of energy I had as a vegetarian and as a vegan. It makes sense—not only was I eating more fruits, veggies, and whole grains, but I was no longer eating things that dragged me down. Do you remember a time when you had a big bowl of mac and cheese and afterwards you just wanted to sleep? Now when I eat a big bowl of mac and *vegan* cheese, I don't feel like napping for hours—I feel like going back to whatever I was doing!

Teenage rebellion! I do *not* advocate going vegan because it makes you different or special or a rebel, but come on. Those kids with blue hair who think they're so punk and question society? If they're not vegan, they're still buying into a huge part of society without a single question or complaint. Try rejecting a notion deeply held by the majority of the world by changing the way you live your day-to-day life and the way you think. Vegans are the real rebels!

Good AR-Related Songs

(or at least with lyrics you can connect to veganism)

"Clever Meals" by Tegan & Sara. For when you don't understand why more people don't care, but are glad that, at the very least, *you* care. "I'm quite sure we'll find one another / In a place that's better than this / A time filled with us / And we send up our shooting stars and comets / Yes we make our little gestures / Yeah we make our little comments"

"You Think It's a Joke" by Goldfinger. A nice angry song when you're completely frustrated with people just laughing off things that are really important. "You think it's a joke / I find no reason why I should laugh at you / You think it's a joke / to take advantage of the life that supports you"

"Walk Away" by Goldfinger. When it gets tiring dealing with stupid people and you want to pitch the whole giving-a-damn thing, this song helps you remember that you, yes, you are the voice of the voiceless and restores your hope in, um, everything. "I don't believe this shit / I know I can make things better / I know it'll take some work / But I'm not afraid of the dirt"

"Free Me" by Goldfinger. What an animal might sing to us. The music video to this song is the only one that's ever made me cry. "I am built like my father was / I've done nothing wrong / So free me / I just want to feel what life should be"

"Meat Is Murder" by the Smiths. A classic that will send chills up your spine and really get you thinking about how barbaric people are. "Heifer whines could be human cries / Closer comes the screaming knife / This beautiful creature must die / This beautiful creature must die / A death for no reason / And death for no reason is murder"

"Be Healthy" by Dead Prez. Eating plants is healthizzle, eating animals is not, and that's all there is to it, homeslice. "I don't eat no meat / no dairy no sweets / Only ripe vegetables, fresh fruit and whole wheat / I'm from the old school / My household smell like soul food, bro"

"Alright" by Supergrass. For the good happy times, when you realize that you *are* making a difference, when you're sitting around eating Tofutti Cuties with your vegan friends. "We are strange in our world / But are young, we run green / Keep our teeth nice and clean / See our friends, see the sights, feel alright"

"Black Masks and Gasoline" by Rise Against. Good. Angry. Not explicitly AR but it's difficult *not* to connect the song to AR when you're vegan. What's not to like? "A need for revolution's rising / It comes to the surface, gasping for air / We're not putting up with this planet / For one more day / Much less one more year"

"Apparently, I'm A 'P.C. Fascist' (Because I Care About Both Human and Non-Human Animals)" by Propagandhi.

Amazing. Propagandhi is my best friend. I really can't think of one portion of lyrics to put down because the entire song is fantastic, but I'll try. "I kinda thought we all shared common threads / In that we gravitated here to challenge conventions we've been fed / by a culture that treats creatures like machines / And if you buy that shit then how long 'til it's me / that serves as your commodity?"

"Nailing Descartes to the Wall (Liquid) Meat is Still Murder" by Propagandhi. Best lyrics *evar*. That's evar with an "a" so listen up. Have I mentioned that Propagandhi is the best? This song is really part two of the one above. "You cannot deny that meat is still murder / and dairy is still rape / I'm still as stupid as anyone / but I know my mistakes / I have recognized one form of oppression, now I'll recognize the rest"

"Bohemian Like You" by the Dandy Warhols. This song isn't really about veganism or AR, but it says "vegan" and it's fun, so that's good enough for me. "But if you dig on vegan food / well come over to my work / I'll have 'em cook you something that you really love / 'cuz I like you / And I feel so bohemian like you"

"Vegan Freak Radio Theme Song" by Rat and K@. When was the last time you rocked out to a theme song to anything? That's what I thought. You can download this song at veganfreakradio.com. "When we were kids the bugs and the birds fascinated us / they were just like us / but we were taught to slam the door / it's not cool to feel to much / but some of us break free"

"Liar" by Bikini Kill. "Eat meat / hate blacks / beat your fucking wife / it's all the same thing / deny, you live your life in denial, baby"

Chapter Thirteen: Where Do I Find...

"I hear there's been rumors on the Internets."

—George W. Bush

Whether you're looking for information, vegan friends, or some of the products you read about in Chapter 8, you can find what you're looking for somewhere out there on the wide world of the web.

Learn!

Veganfreaks.org — A blog, blog list, podcast, and forums run by the fine folks behind the Vegan Freaks vegan media empire. Probably the veg website I visit the most. Entries insightful, links helpful, podcast kick-ass.

GoVeg.com — Yeah, it's done by PETA, but it still has some great info on a very broad range of topics, from animal agriculture and the environment to vegan health to why you should be vegan. They actually do a pretty good job of citing their sources and whatnot.

VegCityGuide.com — A comprehensive list of locally run veg*n city guides, with lots of cities represented. Generally you'll have more luck with specific, locally run veg*n guides than broader, nonlocal ones.

VegProductsGuide.com — A guide to vegan product alternatives to meat, pet food, dairy, and all that stuff. Plus, you can see what other veg*ns think of certain products!

Eat!

VegWeb.com is a great resource when you've got some ingredients but aren't sure what to do with them, or when you know there has to be a recipe for something you want to eat but aren't sure where to find it.

VegCooking.com is another good, general recipes site. Like VegWeb, it's exclusively vegan and you can simply search for what you have or what you want to make.

VegGuide.org is a resource for finding veg restaurants and health food stores in your area. Just find your region, state/province, city, and voila, you probably have a new place to eat. Great for travel.

HappyCow.net is similar to VegGuide, but it also has some recipes.

Buy!

VeganEssentials.com — Vegan food, clothes, vitamins, bags, shoes, candles, candy, toiletries/cosmetics, pet food...if you can't find it here I don't know where you can. Warehouse in Wisconsin.

HerbivoreClothing.com — Fabulous tees, totes, stickers, belts, hoodies, buttons, etc. Not just boxy, boring shirts that happen to say something about veganism, but clothes you'd actually wear even if they didn't have vegan messages. Be a well-dressed vegan. Also some books. Storefront in Portland, Oregon.

CosmosVeganShoppe.com — Things to eat. Things to wear. Things to write on. Things to make you smell pretty. Things to give to lucky people. Many, many, many lovely vegan things. Plus, every item has a rating (one cat to five cats), very helpful. Storefront in Atlanta, Georgia.

VeganStore.com — Pangea Vegan Store is from this website. Everything but the kitchen sink. Vegan gift baskets and coats and books, too. Very first store of its kind.

AlternativeOutfitters.com — Vegans need clothes, too. Non-animal bags, belts, shoes, and more. T-shirts and tanks with vegan messages. Some skin-care/hair-care items, too. Woohoo!

MooShoes.com — Wide selection of vegan shoes, belts, bags, wallets, purses, jackets, etc., plus books and videos of the vegan variety. Storefront in New York City.

Befriend!

Meetup.com — find a vegetarian/vegan meetup group in your area (or start one)! I don't know what I would do without my local group. Having a vegan support system is incredibly important. Common meetup group activities are potlucks, restaurant outings, activism events, and more.

VegWeb.com — If you're eighteen or over, you can set up a profile here and find veg*n friends, penpals, etc.

VegSpace.com — Like MySpace but for veg*n folk.

INDEX

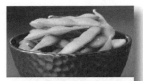

New American Vegan
Vincent Guihan
$17.95 • ISBN: 978-1-60486-079-5

All across North America, people are looking to make better choices, but also eat healthier, more environmentally friendly and, most of all, great tasting food. *New American Vegan* breaks from a steady stream of cookbooks inspired by fusion and California cuisines that put catchy titles and esoteric ingredients first in their efforts to cater to a cosmopolitan taste. Instead, Vincent goes back to his Midwestern roots to play a humble but important role in the reinvention of American cuisine while bringing the table back to the center of American life.

Weaving together small town values, personal stories and 120 great recipes, *New American Vegan* delivers authentically American food that simply has to be tasted to be believed. Recipes range from very basic to the modestly complicated, but always with an eye on creating something that is both beautiful and delicious while keeping it simple. Clear instructions provide step by steps, but also help new cooks find their feet in the kitchen, with a whole chapter devoted just to terms, tools and techniques. With an eye towards improvisation, the book provides a detailed basic recipe that's good as-is, but also provides additional notes that explain how to take each recipe further, to increase flavor, to add drama to the presentation or just how to add a little extra flourish for new cooks and seasoned kitchen veterans.

"Guihan has a knack for infusing bold and fiery seasonings into fresh produce and vegan pantry staples—creating inventive, novel recipes that will inspire and excite the vegan home cook."
—Dreena Burton, author of *Eat, Drink, & Be Vegan*

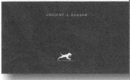

Cook, Eat, Thrive:
Vegan Recipes from Everyday to Exotic
Joy Tienzo
$17.95 • ISBN: 978-1-60486-509-7

In *Cook, Eat, Thrive*, Joy Tienzo encourages you to savor the cooking process while crafting distinctive meals from fresh, flavorful ingredients. Enjoy comfortable favorites. Broaden your culinary horizons with internationally-inspired dishes. Share with friends and family, and create cuisine that allows people, animals, and the environment to fully thrive.

Cook, Eat, Thrive features dishes including:

- Buttermilk Biscuits with Southern Style Gravy
- Earl Grey Carrot Muffins
- Orange Cream Green Smoothie
- Palm Heart Ceviche
- Barbecue Ranch Salad
- Raspberry Chèvre Salad with Champagne Vinaigrette

- Samosa Soup
- Tarte aux Poireaux et Pommes de Terre
- Italian Cornmeal Cake with Roasted Apricots and Coriander Crème Anglaise
- Lavender Rice Pudding Brûlée with Blueberries
- Peanut Butter Shortbread with Concord Grape Sorbet

Inside, you'll find: an extensive equipment and ingredients listing; basics like seitan, non-dairy milks, grains, frozen desserts, and salad dressing; menus for occasions, from Caribbean-inspired garden parties to vegan weddings; practical symbols to let you know if recipes are raw, low fat, soy-free, wheat-free, approachable for non-vegans, and quick fix.

"*Cook, Eat, Thrive* gives vegans the option of choosing exotic and extraordinary recipes for special dinner preparations, or simpler, yet imaginative creations for day to day meal planning. Whether you're looking for everyday vegan fare, or exquisite vegan dining, Tienzo serves it up with culinary flair!"
—Dreena Burton, author of *Eat, Drink, & Be Vegan*

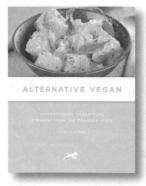

Alternative Vegan:
International Vegan Fare Straight
From the Produce Aisle
Dino Sarma
$17.95 • ISBN: 978-1-60486-508-0

Tofu, seitan, tempeh, tofu, seitan, tempeh ... it seems like so many vegans rely on these products as meat substitutes. Isn't it time to break out of the mold?

Taking a fresh, bold, and alternative approach to vegan cooking without the substitutes, Dino Sarma brings you over 100 fully vegan recipes, many of which draw from his South Asian roots. Sharing his jazz-style approach to cooking, Dino also discusses how you can improvise in your own cooking with simple ingredients and how you can stock your kitchen to prepare simple and delicious vegan meals quickly.

Whether you love tofu, seitan, and tempeh or hate it, *Alternative Vegan* shows you how to let the flavor shine through by cooking simply with fresh ingredients. Dino helps you create mouth-watering dishes such as:
- One-pot meals and big salads: from warming soups, South-Indian uppama, and chipotle garlic risotto to beautiful composed salads
- Basic dishes: using few ingredients but big on flavor, like basic broccoli, demonic mushrooms, or Asian roasted potatoes
- International dishes such as Pakoras, Flautas, Bajji, and Kashmiri Biriyani
- Simple snacks and appetizers like hummus canapes and no-cheese pizzas

Explore your inner chef and get cooking with Dino!

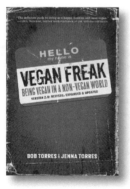

Vegan Freak:
Being Vegan in a Non-Vegan World
Bob & Jenna Torres
$14.95 • ISBN: 978-1-60486-015-3

Going vegan is easy, and even easier if you have the tools at hand to make it work right. In the second edition of this informative and practical guide, two seasoned vegans help you learn to love your inner vegan freak. Loaded with tips, advice, and stories, this book is the key to helping you thrive as a happy, healthy, and sane vegan in a decidedly non-vegan world that doesn't always get what you're about. In this sometimes funny, sometimes irreverent, and sometimes serious guide that's not afraid to tell it like it is, you will:

- find out how to go vegan in three weeks or less with our "cold tofu method"
- discover and understand the arguments for ethical, abolitionist veganism
- learn how to convince family, friends, and others that you haven't joined a vegetable cult by going vegan
- get some advice on dealing with people in your life without creating havoc or hurt feelings
- learn to survive restaurants, grocery stores, and meals with omnivores
- find advice on how to respond when people ask you if you "like, live on apples and twigs."

The first edition has sold over 10,000 copies. In a revised and expanded second edition, *Vegan Freak* is your guide to embracing vegan freakdom.

"Bob and Jenna Torres not only convince you that you have to go vegan today, they also give you what you need to live as a healthy and happy vegan for the rest of your life."
—Gary L. Francione, Distinguished Professor of Law, Rutgers University

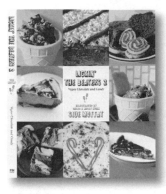

Lickin' the Beaters 2:
Vegan Chocolate and Candy
Siue Moffat
$17.95 • ISBN: 978-1-60486-009-2

The beaters go on—in *Lickin' the Beaters 2*, the second of Siue Moffat's fun vegan dessert cookbooks.

Themed around the duality of desert—an angel on one shoulder and a devil on the other—Siue takes chocolate, candy and even ice creem head-on with quirky illustrations, useful hints, and a handy "Quick Recipe" indicator to make using this book simple and amusing. With an understanding that dessert should be an indulgence, Moffat provides vegan renditions of tantalizing delicacies, both traditional and original.

Recipes include old favorites such as Carmel Corn, Salt Water Taffy, Pralines, Cookies, Cakes and Fudge, as well as some brave new gluten-free recipes like Fabulous Flourless Chocolate Torte and Toll-Free Chocolate Chip cookies.

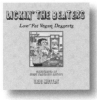

Still Available
Lickin' the Beaters: Low Fat Vegan Desserts
Siue Moffat • $10.95 • ISBN: 978-1-60486-004-7

"A wonderful and delightful collection of recipes that tantalize your tastebuds into thinking you're being decadent and naughty. A real treat for anyone who loves a good dessert."
— Sarah Kramer co-author of *How It All Vegan*

Cook Food:
A Manualfesto for Easy, Healthy, Local Eating
Lisa Jervis
$12.00 • 978-1-60486-073-3

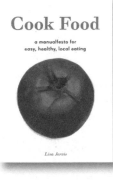

More than just a rousing food manifesto and a nifty set of tools, Cook Food makes preparing tasty, wholesome meals simple and accessible for those hungry for both change and scrumptious fare. If you're used to getting your meals from a package—or the delivery guy—or if you think you don't know how to cook, this is the book for you.

If you want to eat healthier but aren't sure where to start, or if you've been reading about food politics but don't know how to bring sustainable eating practices into your everyday life, *Cook Food* will give you the scoop on how, while keeping your taste buds satisfied. With a conversational, do-it-yourself vibe, a practical approach to everyday cooking on a budget, and a whole bunch of animal-free recipes, *Cook Food* will have you cooking up a storm, tasting the difference, thinking globally and eating locally.

"Overwhelmed by all the politics on your plate? Paralyzed by guilt every time you shop for food? In this swift and delectable guide, Lisa Jervis shows not just how easy it can be to eat with your conscience and with the planet, but also how cheap, how swift, and how delightful it is to feel at home in the kitchen."
— Raj Patel, author of *Stuffed and Starved*

"Thanks to Lisa Jervis for not only distilling such important information into digestible bites, but for putting the theory into practice with excellent and inspiring recipes. Potluck at my place, please!"
— Michelle Tea, author of *Rose of No Man's Land* and *Rent Girl*

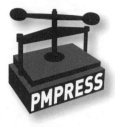

PM Press was founded at the end of 2007 by a small collection of folks with decades of publishing, media, and organizing experience. PM Press co-conspirators have published and distributed hundreds of books, pamphlets, CDs, and DVDs. Members of PM have founded enduring book fairs, spearheaded victorious tenant organizing campaigns, and worked closely with bookstores, academic conferences, and even rock bands to deliver political and challenging ideas to all walks of life. We're old enough to know what we're doing and young enough to know what's at stake.

We seek to create radical and stimulating fiction and non-fiction books, pamphlets, t-shirts, visual and audio materials to entertain, educate, and inspire you. We aim to distribute these through every available channel with every available technology, whether that means you are seeing anarchist classics at our bookfair stalls; reading our latest vegan cookbook at the café; downloading geeky fiction e-books; or digging new music and timely videos from our website.

PM Press is always on the lookout for talented and skilled volunteers, artists, activists, and writers to work with. If you have a great idea for a project or can contribute in some way, please get in touch.

PM Press • PO Box 23912 • Oakland CA 94623
www.pmpress.org

FRIENDS OF PM

These are indisputably momentous times—the financial system is melting down globally and the Empire is stumbling. Now more than ever there is a vital need for radical ideas.

In the three years since its founding—and on a mere shoestring—PM Press has risen to the formidable challenge of publishing and distributing knowledge and entertainment for the struggles ahead. With over 100 releases to date, we have published an impressive and stimulating array of literature, art, music, politics, and culture. Using every available medium, we've succeeded in connecting those hungry for ideas and information to those putting them into practice.

Friends of PM allows you to directly help impact, amplify, and revitalize the discourse and actions of radical writers, filmmakers, and artists. It provides us with a stable foundation from which we can build upon our early successes and provides a much-needed subsidy for the materials that can't necessarily pay their own way. You can help make that happen—and receive every new title automatically delivered to your door once a month—by joining as a Friend of PM Press. And, we'll throw in a free t-shirt when you sign up.

Here are your options:
- $25 a month: Get all books and pamphlets plus 50% discount on all webstore purchases
- $25 a month: Get all CDs and DVDs plus 50% discount on all webstore purchases
- $40 a month: Get all PM Press releases plus 50% discount on all webstore purchases
- $100 a month: Superstar—Everything plus PM merchandise, free downloads, and 50% discount on all webstore purchases

For those who can't afford $25 or more a month, we're introducing Sustainer Rates at $15, $10, and $5. Sustainers get a free PM Press t-shirt and a 50% discount on all purchases from our website.

Your Visa or Mastercard will be billed once a month, until you tell us to stop. Or until our efforts succeed in bringing the revolution around. Or the financial meltdown of Capital makes plastic redundant. Whichever comes first.